Addictive Disorders in Arctic Climates: Theory, Research and Practice at the Novosibirsk Institute

Addictive Disorders in Arctic Climates: Theory, Research and Practice at the Novosibirsk Institute

Bernard Segal, PhD
Caesar Korolenko, MD
Editors

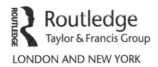

Routledge
Taylor & Francis Group

LONDON AND NEW YORK

First Published 1990 by The Haworth Press, Inc.

Published 2016 by Routledge
2 Park Square, Milton Park, Abingdon, Oxfordshire OX14 4RN
711 Third Avenue, New York, NY 10017

First issued in paperback 2016

Routledge is an imprint of the Taylor and Francis Group, an informa business

Addictive Disorders in Arctic Climates: Theory, Research and Practice at the Novosibirsk Institute has also been published as *Drugs & Society*, Volume 4, Numbers 3/4 1990.

Library of Congress Cataloging-in-Publication Data

Addictive disorders in arctic climates : theory, research and practice at the Novosibirsk Institute /
Bernard Segal, Caesar Korolenko, editors,

    p. cm.

"Has also been published as Drugs & society, volume 4, numbers 3/4, 1990" —T.p. verso.
Includes papers translated from the Russian.
ISBN 1-56024-036-9

    1. Alcoholism— Arctic regions. 2. Alcoholism— Alaska. 3. Alcoholism — Siberia (R.S.F.S.R.) 4. Novosibirskii gosudarstvennyi meditsinskii institut. Dept, of Psychiatry and Medical Psychology. I. Segal, Bernard. II. Korolenko, TS. P. (TSezar' Petrovich)

    [DNLM: 1. Novosibirskii gosudarstvennyi meditsinskii institut. Dept, of Psychiatry and Medical Psychology. 2. Alcoholism. 3. Cold Climate.]
RC564.75.A68A33 1990
616.86T09113-dc20
DNLM/DLC
for Library of Congress   90-4611
    CIP

ISBN 13: 978-1-138-98828-6 (pbk)
ISBN 13: 978-1-56024-036-5 (hbk)

Addictive Disorders in Arctic Climates: Theory, Research and Practice at the Novosibirsk Institute

CONTENTS

ALL HAWORTH BOOKS & JOURNALS
ARE PRINTED ON CERTIFIED
ACID-FREE PAPER

ABOUT THE EDITORS

Bernard Segal, PhD, is a professor of Health Sciences at the University of Alaska, Anchorage. Dr. Segal began at the University of Alaska in 1977 as Training Coordinator within the Center for Alcohol and Addiction Studies. He was named the Center's Director in 1979 and continued in that role until January 1989, when he returned to full time research and teaching.

His research interest is in the psychosocial correlates of drug-taking behavior. A recipient of both federal and state grants, his research had led to two books, numerous publications and presentations, and to collaboration with researchers in other countries. He has been to Israel and Japan as a visiting professor, and has been invited to the Soviet Union, where he is currently involved in a collaborative project with alcohol researchers in Novosibirsk, Siberia.

After earning a doctorate in clinical psychology from the University of Oklahoma in 1967, Dr. Segal taught at the University of Rhode Island for several years before becoming Director of the Psychological Center and of Clinical Training at Murray State University in Kentucky. During this time, he was also a police psychologist at the Murray Police Department.

Caesar Korolenko, MD, is Director of the Department of Psychiatry and Medical Psychology at the Novosibirsk Medical Institute, Novosibirsk, Siberia, USSR. He is responsible for the teaching of psychiatry to beginning and advanced medical students and for the treatment of patients with addictive disorders. He leads a research team within his unit that has studied the problem of alcoholism in Siberia. Although he has published extensively within the USSR, this is his first opportunity to share his work outside the Soviet Union.

Preface

In January, 1983, as part of a delegation that visited Novosibirsk, Siberia, USSR, the home of The Siberian Branch of The Soviet Academy of Medical Sciences, I had the pleasure of meeting Dr. Caesar P. Korolenko, Director, Department of Psychiatry and Medical Psychology, Novosibirsk Medical Institute. His being extremely fluent in English, together with a mutual agreeable approach to understanding alcoholism and other forms of drug-taking behavior, helped us to establish quickly a close personal and professional relationship.

At that time a beginning was made toward establishing cooperative Siberian-American studies of addictive disorders. This collaborative effort was facilitated through The Siberian Branch of the USSR Academy of Medical Sciences. Dr. Yuri Nikitin, Deputy Director of the Siberian Branch, AMS, and Director of International Relations, was instrumental in helping this arrangement to mature. Dr. Igor G. Ursov, Director of the Novosibirsk Medical Institute, also contributed to this relationship by providing support for Dr. Korolenko to participate in this collaborative effort.

The purpose of this collaboration was to focus on common and specific characteristics of addictive disorders in two similar arctic and subarctic regions (Alaska and Siberia) in order to develop an understanding of the etiology of such disorders, and to work toward establishing effective intervention, treatment and prevention strategies relevant to both regions.

Although a collaborative relationship was formed between the University of Alaska Anchorage and The Siberian Branch of The Soviet Academy of Medical Sciences in 1983, it was not until the fall of 1988 that this relationship began to develop fully, leading to expanded collaborative research efforts which encompassed broad-based biomedical research programs between Siberian and Alaskan researchers.

xi

In November, 1988, through the efforts of Dr. Yuri Nikitin, a delegation of researchers from the University of Alaska returned to Novosibirsk to establish contact with our Siberian counterparts. Dr. Sven Ebbesson, Head of the Alaska Delegation, worked with Dr. Nikitin to develop a plan for cooperative research.

During this visit I had the opportunity to renew my friendship in person with Dr. Korolenko. The intervening years did not dampen our enthusiasm to work together, and we viewed this new occasion as a chance to move ahead rapidly. Our fundamental approach to understanding alcoholism and substance abuse, and our research interests, remained extremely similar. Dr. Korolenko introduced me to his colleagues in the Department of Psychiatry and Medical Psychology, and together we discussed mutual concerns about alcohol- and drug-related problems, and other issues. This exchange was extremely frank and candid, and I was impressed by their efforts.

As a result of what I learned from this group of research-practitioners (N. L. Botchkareva, MD, V. Yu. Zavjalov, MD, A. S. Timofeeva, MD, L. F. Perekrjostova, MD, T. A. Donskih, MD, and A. Dragun, MD), I asked Dr. Korolenko if manuscripts reporting on their research could be prepared for citation in a special edition of *Drugs & Society*. This issue, as I envisioned it, was to be devoted to reporting the research that he and his team of research-practitioners were conducting. I believed that this special issue would be worthwhile because it would provide a unique opportunity to learn about the interesting perspectives on addiction studies practiced by the Novosibirsk group.

There was unanimous agreement to have their research published in *Drugs & Society*, and Dr. Korolenko assumed responsibility to coordinate the manuscript from Novosibirsk. Although they were originally written in Russian, he translated them into literal English. These articles represented the first Siberian-American cooperative effort between addiction researchers in Novosibirsk and Alaska.

In November, 1989, Dr. Korolenko and a delegation of Siberian scientists visited Alaska to further the collaborative projects derived from the earlier meeting in Novosibirsk. He and I spent 10 days absolutely "glued" to my computer taking his literal translation of the manuscripts and working to refine their translation. What appears in this issue is the result of this collaborative effort.

The five reports are presented as an introduction to and overview of the perspectives on addictive disorders held by the research-practitioners at the Department of Psychiatry and Medical Psychology, Novosibirsk Medical Institute. The focus is primarily on their philosophy and on reports of their research; methodology was not emphasized. The intent, at this time in our joint venture, is not to focus on procedure, but to provide an introduction to their research approaches, and to review the implications of the findings.

Therefore this series of articles contain a general discussion of attitudes toward the problem of alcoholism, epidemiology of addictive disorders, classification of addictive behaviors, attitudes toward treatment and prevention, and a description of clinical symptoms of alcoholism and psychological disorders and their progression in both men and women. In each of these studies the concept of addictive behavior is expressed, a concept specific to practitioners and researchers at the Novosibirsk Department of Psychiatry.

This concept is, in many aspects, different from traditional attitudes about addiction held by many Soviet and even American practitioners. Addictive behavior is perceived by the Novosibirsk group as a subcondition of a broader condition of deviant behavior, and as a complex problem which includes not only biological factors, but also environmental, social, psychological, cultural, economic, and developmental elements. Special attention in these papers is given to describing the psychological factors involved in the formation of an addictive disorder, specifically alcoholism.

These reports, however, do have limitations. For example, when citations of research studies are made there are reduced discussions about the methods of data collection and about the samples studied. While this limitation is a short-coming based on contemporary standards for reporting research, part of it resulted from my urging to focus on primarily communicating perspectives on addictive disorders rather than stressing methodological procedures. The manuscripts were thus prepared with the idea of presenting theoretical perspectives and limiting discussions of methodology. The responsibility thus rests with me for the style of the manuscripts, and not with the authors.

While some readers may interpret this deficiency as a weakness which precludes the utility of the research reports, I made the decision, after consultation with some members of the editorial board, and others,[1] to go ahead and publish them because of the importance of conveying what is happening in one part of the USSR with respect to addiction studies. Moreover, because of time deadlines, and difficulty in rapid communication between Alaska and Novosibirsk, I believe that to have attempted to expand the manuscripts to account more fully for the methodology would have led to an extremely lengthy delay of over a year before this issue would have been ready for publication. I assumed that it was more important to get these articles into print, as imperfect as they might be perceived to be, in order to share in the spirit of "Glasnost." It was also important, I believe, to use this issue to open a dialogue with our Soviet counterparts, leading to a greater exchange of information. Subsequent reports, therefore, will be more precise, and also include findings from joint research, as well as contain reviews of how the Novosibirsk research compares with research findings from other studies conducted in cold regions, or from those pursuing a biopsychosocial approach to the study of addictive disorders.

In all, I believe these papers provide a rare opportunity to examine the theories and practice of a small group of medical-research practitioners in Novosibirsk. It is anticipated that they will inspire American researchers and practitioners to learn more about research in the USSR, and to determine what implications their work has for American researchers and practitioners.

I would also like to acknowledge the valued assistance of Marguerite Lambert, for her work in typing the original manuscripts, and helping to edit the final drafts.

Bernard Segal, PhD

---

1. I would like to acknowledge the assistance of Dr. Joseph Westermeyer, University of Oklahoma School of Medicine, and Dr. G. Alan Marlazz, University of Washington, for their review of the manuscripts and editorial suggestions.

Introduction

Bernard Segal, PhD

As noted in the preface, these articles represent reports of research from a group of research-practitioners at the Department of Psychiatry, Novosibirsk, Siberia, USSR.

In the first report, "A Review of the Problem of Alcoholism in Siberia," by Korolenko and Botchkareva, they convey that an important part of their effort to understand drinking behavior involves the study of the interaction among specific ecological, demographical, and medical-social factors. They do not separate the problem of alcoholism from this context. They approach drinking as a problem involving a complex interaction among social, economic, cultural and educative factors. Focusing on only one of these elements without consideration of the others, they state, will not help in developing a comprehensive understanding of alcoholism.

An important implication that the Siberian research has, especially for Alaskan researchers, is that we have to orient ourselves to focus more extensively on understanding how the relationship between adjustment to living in an extreme geo-climatic environment and social-psychological change contribute to the development of psychological and physical dependence to alcohol. Is, for example, the onset of alcohol-related problems more accelerated among newcomers when compared to longer-term residents of cold regions. Another important implication, with respect to Alaska Natives, or other aboriginal people, is the following question: To what extent is the onset of alcoholism a function of psychological adaptation resulting from cultural change.

The second article, "Clinical-Psychological Approaches to Alcoholism: Multiple Versions of Alcohol Dependence," by V. Yu. Zavjalov, presents a philosophical overview of issues that practitioners and theorists continue to struggle with. In this carefully conceived paper Dr. Zavjalov address what Dr. Joseph Westermeyer describes as "a current problem in alcoholism treatment across nations and cultures . . . [which is the issue of] how individualized should assessment and treatment for alcoholism be? Should the 'all alcoholics are the same' strategy to the assessment and treatment of alcoholism be replaced by a more individualized approach. (J. Westermeyer, personal communication, July 25, 1989.)

Dr. Zavjalov, who advocates an individualized approach, presents a well referenced discussion of both Soviet and American literature in support of his theoretical view.

In the following presentation titled "Social-Psychological Aspects of Drinking by Youth and Adults," by Timofeeva and Perekrjostova, there is a discussion of four developmental stages they postulate that are related to teenage alcoholism. Although it is not stated clearly in the article, the evolvement of the four stages were based on research studies carried out at the Novosibirsk Medical Institute. Rather than describing the research, these authors have chosen to discuss the implications of their research in the form of describing what they believe are developmental stages involved in the onset of teenage alcoholism. The particular value of this article is that it provides a perspective on how the study of teenage alcoholism is being approached at the Novosibirsk Medical Institute.

The paper, "Addictive Behavior in Women: A Theoretical Perspective," by Korolenko and Donskih, presents a comprehensive review of both applied and theoretical perspectives. Based on a synthesis of research studies carried out by Korolenko and his colleagues, it presents an extensive summary of their findings. The details of the specific research studies, such as a description of the sampling method and the sources of data, however, were not clearly delineated, nor were details of the questionnaire and interview process provided. Although this lack of information may preclude replication of this study, the information conveyed should nevertheless help to establish a theoretical base to begin to develop similar research. Moreover, Korolenko and Donskih, in their effort to convey the essence of their research, emphasized the findings and implications of their research to a greater extent than the specific methodology.

The last article, "The 'Rapid Course of Development' of Early

Alcoholism in Young People," by A. Dragun, presents an interesting review of the approach to alcoholism pursued by the Novosibirsk group. Two specific areas of study are emphasized. One is the study of whether there is a difference in the length of onset of what may be described as alcoholism which involves physical dependency (e.g., Jellineck's concept of Gamma Alcoholism), between long term inhabitants of a region, such as Northern Siberia, and newcomers to the northernmost region, who have to adjust to changes in geo-climatic and social conditions. The second area of investigation concerns the symptoms of alcoholism itself. The question first asked is whether there is a more rapid onset of alcohol-related problems among newcomers compared to long-term inhabitants (of the central part of Siberia)? Then the question of what form these symptoms take arises. The Novosibirsk group found that new comers not only developed alcoholism earlier than longer-term inhabitants of the middle region, but that they also showed different clinical symptoms. The process of early onset of alcoholism was described as the *Rapid Development of Alcoholism* syndrome. The essential element of the clinical symptoms associated with Rapid Development of Alcoholism was that they showed high levels of stress and frequently drank large amounts of alcohol quickly leading to deep intoxicated states. Much of their drinking was motivated to reduce stress. The findings from this research have important implications concerning the etiology of alcoholism, and provide an interesting perspective to facilitate further research.

Following the reports of research from Novosibirsk are a series of reviews. The first is a general overview of the approach taken by the Novosibirsk group by Dr. Dan Lettieri, formerly of the National Institute on Drug Abuse and the National Institute on Alcohol Abuse and Alcoholism. His comments center on comparing the work in Novosibirsk with contemporary American approaches.

Subsequent to his review is a progression of reviews of each of the Novosibirsk articles from faculty of the University of Michigan Substance Abuse Center. These reviews, coordinated by Dr. Frederick B. Glaser, Director of the Substance Abuse Center, provide a diversity of views. Some of the Siberian papers evoked special interest, especially "Clinical-Psychological Approaches to Alcoholism: Multiple Versions of Alcohol Dependence," by V. Yu.

Zavjalov, and thus were reviewed by two or more faculty members. These reviews provide a perspective on the Siberian papers by American research-practitioners which facilitates a comparison with contemporary thinking and practices in the United States.

I would like to extend my appreciation to Dr. Glaser for having undertaken the coordination of the reviews, and for his two contributions. I would also like to thank the other reviewers (J. Brower, MD, Thomas P. Bresford, MD, T. E. Dielman, PhD, Beth Glover Reed, PhD, and Edith S. Lisansky-Gomberg, PhD) for their contributions.

In summary, I believe that the value of this issue is that it introduces the audience, for the first time, to the interesting and challenging research pursued by a group of Soviet research-practitioners struggling in Novosibirsk, Siberia, to deal with the problem of alcoholism in a rapidly changing society. Their work is both progressive and insightful. We can benefit from their endeavors (thus my haste to share their work with you), and as barriers come down between our two nations, we will all benefit from the exchange of information that will follow.

A Review of the Problem
of Alcoholism in Siberia

C. P. Korolenko, MD
N. L. Botchkareva, MD

INTRODUCTION

Scientific progress and technical development in societies are related to the development of resources and to population growth in new regions. This development, in the case of Siberia, occurred under such extraordinary conditions that it exerted a strong influence on the people in the region, both newcomers and Native Siberians. These extraordinary conditions encompass both natural and anthropogenic factors, which appear in connection with industrial development, or which can result from a combination of climatic-meteorological and anthropogenic influences.

A method of measuring climatic conditions has been developed by Rakita and Klimovitch (1974), and is known as the *coefficient-of-general-discomfort-of-climate*. This coefficient takes into account such factors as temperatures below $-30°$ C, stormy winds, heavy snowfall, rainstorms, and other climatic conditions.

Siberia's climate is diverse, but as a whole is characterized by severity. In the southern regions of western and eastern Siberia, the coefficient-of-general-discomfort-of-climate exceeds that found in the central regions of Russia by a factor of two or three. The closer to the north, the higher the coefficient. In the tundra area of Siberia the coefficient is five to seven times higher than in the central re-

C. P. Korolenko and N. L. Botchkareva are affiliated with the Department of Psychiatry, Novosibirsk Medical Institute.

gion of Russia. In the Tajmyr Peninsula, where a series of studies were conducted (see Korolenko, 1978), minimal temperatures of $-52°$ C are present, and winds of 40M per second were common.

The influence of continental and extracontinental climates are combined with considerable oscillations of atmospheric pressure, and in the far north the situation is aggravated by unusual photoperiodicity (periods of polar nights and days). Climatic conditions are also significantly affected by industrial and municipal pollution. These climatic factors, when linked with the psychological aspects of living in extreme conditions (e.g., the impact on sensory processes and different forms of hyperstimulation), together with an increase in lifespan, all contribute to create high levels of stress.

These climatic conditions are not extreme for northern aboriginal people as these indigenous people have adapted to it over a long evolutionary period. But during the last few decades Siberian Natives have been influenced by such factors as acculturation stress and urbanization, especially those who migrate to newly established cities in the north.

Siberian industrial development, particularly in its northern regions, has been connected with a large in-migration of people from other climatic regions, and from rural areas. These people not only had to adapt to extreme climatic conditions, but to new social and psychological factors inherent to living in the north. The adaptation process has also been affected by the body's ability to change to meet new environmental conditions. Psychological adaptation is particularly vulnerable because people are not immediately ready to adjust to such extreme climatic and geographical changes.

When subjected to such extreme geo-climatic conditions, and when having to adapt to a new social environment as well, psychological adaptation can be impaired and psychological distress can be experienced. This stress can be the first symptoms of a possible severe psychological disorder. Failure in psychological adaptation can also cause changes in biological systems, and if timely intervention does not occur negative consequences can develop, such as illnesses of psychophysiological adaptation.

A HISTORICAL PERSPECTIVE

When reviewing drinking-related problems in Siberia, it is important to take into consideration that during the past two to three decades (1950s to the 1980s), Siberia became a large industrial region. The rate of industrial development, settling of new territories, and the migration of hundreds of thousands of people, resulted in specific ecological, demographical, and medical-social problems. The problem of alcoholism cannot be separated from this context, and has to be understood as a problem involving a complex interaction among social, economic, cultural and educative factors. Overcoming alcoholism, however, cannot be achieved through treatment alone, but also has to involve changes in public opinion regarding alcohol, effective organization and coordination of treatment facilities (narcological centers), and social and economic change. In the last decade narcological services, ambulatory (outpatient) centers, hospital treatment wards and industrial clinics were significantly increased. As treatment and intervention services increased, a corresponding increase was observed in patients diagnosed as alcoholic. The morbidity of alcoholism increased more than 8 times since 1961. This high rate of alcoholism in Siberia reflects, on the one hand, an increase in the ability to diagnose alcoholism and, on the other hand, represents the increased rate of alcohol consumption that took place in Siberia during the period of rapid social and economic change.

The number of diagnosed cases and morbidity of alcoholism before 1975, when clinical facilities began to improve their diagnosis of alcoholism, rose more than 10 percent per year. After 1975, the rate decreased to about 4 percent per year. The advances in treatment and efforts at prevention helped to stabilize the index of morbidity. This change was accompanied by a decrease in alcohol psychosis from 15 percent in the 1970s, to 5 percent in the 1980s among alcoholic patients. The rate for diagnosis of psychological dependence on alcohol was much lower than physical dependence (about 12%) because of difficulties encountered in the diagnosis of early symptoms of alcoholism. Currently, women constitute 10-12 percent of all cases diagnosed as alcoholic, and teenagers are represented in 3-4 percent of all cases.

In 1985 the USSR enacted a special anti-alcohol decree which was directed at reducing alcohol consumption. This decree affected the production of alcohol, and changed the administrative, legal and medical measures involved in treating alcohol problems in society. After four years some positive effects have been observed. Most important, attitudes toward drinking have changed in that people became more aware of the adverse affects of alcohol, and the social pressure for people to drink was reduced. One positive result of this change was that it helped to lower the incidence of alcohol-related problems because people at risk for development of alcoholism reduced their overall alcohol consumption. Another positive affect was a reduction in alcohol-related deaths. Work productivity increased, and family situations improved. The prevalence of alcohol psychosis between 1986 and 1987 decreased by a factor of two when compared to statistics prior to 1985.

In contrast to these positive gains, the decrease in availability of alcohol resulted in: (1) a considerable increase in home-brewing, (2) higher levels of intoxication among those who continued to drink, (3) an increase in production of illicit ("bootleg") whiskey, (4) an increase in consumption of commercial products containing alcohol, and (5) an increase in the use of other mind-altering substances, such as tranquilizers, hashish, anti-Parkinson drugs, and inhalant substances.

These adverse effects are connected with the interpretation by local officials of the Government's Decree as a prohibition law. Local authorities took it upon themselves to stress prohibition without taking into account the effects that a reduction in availability in alcohol would bring. Prohibition in the absence of the development of a multi-level prevention program is insufficient to totally reduce consumption. It is important to realize that alcoholism is the product of a complex interaction among alcohol availability, psychosocial processes, and economic and cultural factors, as well as education. Focusing on only one of these elements without consideration of the others will only partly help in dealing with the problem of alcoholism.

PSYCHOEMOTIONAL TENSION AND DRINKING

Two interrelated projects were undertaken by Korolenko and his colleagues at the Novosibirsk Medical Institute to study the relationship between psychomotor tension and drinking. The first consisted of an attempt to identify specific adjustment problems among 1200 men between 20 and 49 years of age with different lengths of time of living in the far north (Korolenko & Botchkareva, 1982). A particular emphasis of the study was to establish the occurrence of the *psychoemotional tension syndrome*. The basic clinical manifestation of this syndrome consists of different degrees of anxiety, ranging from mild free-floating to severe forms. Other symptoms associated with this syndrome are increased agitation, a deterioration in ability to concentrate, and a loss in work-time. An important aspect of this research was to determine the relationship between the psychoemotional tension syndrome and drinking behavior. In-depth psychological interviews and testing, and physiological studies (e.g., blood pressure, EKG, GSR, and neurological evaluations), were also conducted on all 1200 men.

The second investigation consisted of an in-depth study (e.g., Rosenzwing Picture Frustration Test, MMPI, and several measures of adaptive behavior), of 260 men, also between 20 to 49 years, who were interviewed every six months during the first three years of their residence in the north.

It was found that among these 260 men, 200 showed signs of protracted symptoms of psychoemotional tension. These 200 men were then studied over a three year period, being evaluated every six months. The results of this investigation revealed that six months, and between 18 and 24 months (after arrival), were the periods of highest risk for development of a state of psychoemotional tension. A follow-up study of these men found that after three years, 30 percent[1] showed reduction of symptoms without treatment. Nineteen percent were identified as experiencing various forms of psychosomatic illness, including neurosis and arterial hypertonia. Twenty percent revealed some form of addictive behav-

---

1. All figures have been rounded to the nearest whole.

ior, including symptoms of psychological and physical alcohol dependence.

A subsequent study of another cohort of 500 men between the ages of 20 and 59 years (including 300 newcomers), who were diagnosed as alcoholic, found that 100 men were Natives and that 100 were inhabitants of Siberia's middle region. These men were studied to determine the relationship between external influences (i.e., geo-climatic factors) and drinking behavior. Based on responses to special questionnaires, psychological and environmental factors were identified as contributing to either the appearance of or to increases in drinking behavior. Some researchers (Jellinek, 1960; Segal, 1988) consider social and psychological factors as fundamental in the development of alcoholism. In regions where geo-climatic factors are extreme, psycho-social behavior may be directly influenced by external conditions, and thus drinking may be related to a combination of both psychosocial and geo-climatic factors.

Forty percent of the newcomers revealed signs of psychological dependence to alcohol before having arrived in the north. Most of these men were observed to drink more frequently or more chronically during their first year in their new environment, resulting in the onset of alcoholic psychosis. Forty-three percent reported that they attributed the increase in their drinking to a state of inner uneasiness and anxiety and psychological discomfort, which they related to polar nights, polar days, oscillations of atmospheric pressure, and to significant changes in the weather. Of these men, twenty-three percent reported that alcohol contributed to family conflict, 15 percent indicated that they drank as a function of drinking patterns already established in the community, 10 percent noted that they drank because of a deterioration in their social and living conditions, 5 percent stated that they drank more because they had more money, and 4 percent reported that they drank when alcohol was available during their work day, such as while working in a place where alcohol was part of the industrial process.

Twenty-one percent of the people who did not misuse alcohol before arriving in their new environment reported that a subjective unpleasant emotional state was a cause for their beginning to drink. Twenty percent of these indicated that an increase in their drinking was connected with worsening economic conditions. Twenty-one percent stated that either family conflicts over money, household keeping problems, or child rearing problems contributed to their drinking. Twenty-one percent associated the negative influence of their environment with their increase in drinking. Ten percent indicated that their misuse of alcohol was related to drinking in the family, and 7 percent linked their contact with alcohol to their workplace.

Among newcomers, social-psychological factors such as being isolated from family, from former friends, teachers, and from other significant people in their lives, were also significant factors related to the onset of stress. Their former environment was perceived as being more free, which they associated with a feeling that less demands were made of them. They felt that their increased use of alcohol in their new environment was not a problem, and was consistent with the level of drinking taking place around them.

Such situations were typical not only for people who migrated to the north, but also for people who migrated to other regions of the country. This condition was especially typical in Siberia during the past two or three decades in regions where industrial development proceeded rapidly. These attitudes may thus be connected to the effects of moving from villages to towns and to cities.

Another effect of this rapid transition and increased migration was a change in traditional village drinking habits among Siberian Natives. Formerly, drinking was largely connected with special occasions such as wedding celebrations, holidays and festive events. Heavy drinking was permitted during these times, but tended to remain restricted to these occasions. People who consumed alcohol excessively outside of these occasions were considered to be irresponsible, lazy, and as setting a bad example for others. This style of behavior, drinking large doses of alcohol, persevered in the new environment, but without the former restriction to special occasions. The risk for problem drinking became especially high for first and second generation Native Siberian migrants because they never fully adapted to the new urbanized culture.

The study of northern aboriginal people indicated that formation of alcoholism was stimulated by such factors as acculturation stress, disintegration of tribal and family relations and traditional drinking patterns, urbanization, adverse influence of drinking by parents, relatives, and friends, conflict situations at home and in the work place, psychological factors, such as poor self-esteem and identity conflicts, and inability to utilize free-time effectively. Unlike the newcomers, the leading factors contributing to the development of alcoholism among the aboriginal people of the north, who were well adapted to the geo-climatic conditions of the region, were an interaction of social-psychological and biological factors.

Alcohol dependency was only one of the possible forms of deviant behavior. Juvenile delinquency, for example, also increased. Among the newcomers to the north, drinking was associated with changes in emotional states, related to geographic acclimatization. Alcohol, in these cases, was used as a remedy to self-medicate a reduction in one's state of psychoemotional tension.

. A comparison of the onset of alcoholism among newcomers and long-term inhabitants of the middle Siberian region, indicated that the newcomers showed a more rapid onset of different alcoholism-related symptoms than the traditional inhabitants. Some of the early symptoms that were most prominent among the newcomers were psychological dependence, loss of control, withdrawal symptoms, alcoholic amnesia, and reverse tolerance.

A detailed examination of the differences between newcomers and long-term inhabitants of the middle region of Siberia showed that psychological dependence to alcohol in newcomers developed after 2.1 years following their misuse of alcohol. The long-term inhabitants showed psychological dependence after 3.2 years. The newcomers also showed some psychological peculiarities. Most apparent was a relationship between a need to drink and the impact of geo-climatic factors. Additionally, newcomers showed rapid development of loss of control as a symptom of physical dependence to alcohol. Among Siberian Natives, loss of control often appeared without a history of a lengthy period of alcohol misuse, and appeared to be associated with biological factors such as differences in alcohol metabolism.

The average time for the onset of alcohol withdrawal symptoms was also shorter for newcomers, and was much more severe than found in cases among long term non-Native inhabitants of the middle region. For example, seizures appeared more frequently (28%)

among newcomers who experienced withdrawal symptoms than among typical long-term resident alcoholic patients with withdrawal symptoms. Seizures occurred three times more often among newcomers than Siberian Natives. These seizures were not found to be connected with brain trauma, severe infections, or other toxic reactions.

A decrease of alcohol tolerance, as a sign of change in alcohol reactivity, developed earlier in the northern areas than in the middle regions, as was comparable among newcomers and Natives. Alcohol palimpsests also appeared more rapidly among both groups. Both groups also showed a rapid development of drinking bouts.

The northern Siberian Natives took slightly longer to develop alcohol symptoms than newcomers. The Native group also showed atypical forms of inebriate behavior, psychological symptoms and psychical dependency. Part of the symptom formation could be attributable to the unique influences of their specific cultural attitudes and behaviors. Their manifested symptoms, therefore, would differ from alcoholic behaviors typically manifested among newcomers, who expressed more traditional attitudes and behaviors.

SUMMARY

In conclusion, the overall results of our research has shown that the process of adaptation to an extreme geo-climatic environment, together with having to adjust to social-psychological changes, contributes to the development of psychological and physical dependence to alcohol. It was noted that the onset of alcohol-related problems was accelerated among newcomers when compared to long-term residents of Siberia's middle region. Among Siberian Natives, it was observed that significant contributing factors in the onset of alcoholism involved disorders of psychological adaptation resulting from cultural change.

In general, the prevalence of alcoholism is higher in Siberia than in western parts of the USSR. A high rate of industrialization, active population migration, loss of traditional values concerning alcohol, and the trend toward urbanization, have all contributed to the increase in alcoholism observed in Siberia. Efforts at prevention have to be adjusted to conform to the types of problems found in different regions. In the northern part of Siberia, where extreme climatic conditions are present, timely intervention to eliminate emotional distress that occurs in the process of adaptation in newcomers is important. For Northern Siberian Natives, special attention must be concentrated in helping them to overcome acculturation stress, to preserve the unique aspects of their culture, and to realistically learn about how alcohol impacts their culture and health.

It is also essential to identify biological and psychological markers associated with the risk of alcoholism, and develop programs that educate the public about various aspects of alcohol problems. It is also important for health providers, especially the medical community and policy makers, to develop a variety of treatment approaches and not limit themselves to a singular way of viewing alcoholism. Without flexibility in approaching the problem the treatment will not be responsive to the patient's needs. If proper intervention is not accomplished, the patient will then go on to establish a stronger defense system which will make it more difficult to intervene. In the north, where a complex interaction between physical, biological, psychological and social elements are involved in the development of alcoholism, treatment and prevention strategies are needed that address these factors singularly and in relation to each other. This need is especially critical for industries' response to alcohol-related problems.

LIST OF REFERENCES

Jellinek, E. (1960). *The disease concept of alcoholism*. Highland Park, NJ: Hillhouse Press.

Korolenko, C. P. (1978). *Psychophysiology of men under extreme conditions*. Novosibirsk, USSR: Science Press.

Korolenko, C. P., & Bochkareva, N. L. (1982). *Peculiarities of certain exogenic intoxications under northern conditions*. Novosibirsk, USSR: Science Press.

Rakita, S. A., & Klimovich, M. V. (1974). *Climatic areas in the north of the USSR*.

Segal, B. (1988) *Drugs and Behavior*. New York: Gardner Press.

Clinical-Psychological Approaches to Alcoholism: Multiple Versions of Alcohol Dependence

V. Yu. Zavjalov, MD

INTRODUCTION:
A NEW POSITION FOR TACKLING AN OLD PROBLEM – A REVIEW OF THEORETICAL PERSPECTIVE ON ALCOHOLISM

The most popular, the "most official," concept of alcoholism in the Soviet Union is the "clinical-psychiatric-oriented" model of chronic alcoholism, which is accepted as doctrine. Until now, the term "chronic alcoholism" referred to the last stage in a continuum of drinking which extends from "ordinary life drinking" [social drinking], to heavy "systematic drinking," and then to alcoholism. Classical psychiatry tends to expound this viewpoint, which is based on a nosological approach and strict clinical thinking. Within this framework the disease concept of alcoholism has been viewed as a definite and "ossified" progressive disease which has a predictable onset and specific consequences, including different problems, such as social and psychological difficulties, all of which are related to alcohol consumption. According to this clinical scheme, labeled in the 1980s as "unitary stereotype of alcoholic disease" (Bekhtcl, 1986), alcoholism is described as progressing only one way – to the final stage of "alcoholic degradation" and to "alcoholic dementia," and the more rapid the onset of the course of the disease, the greater the personality disorganization.

V. Yu. Zavjalov is affiliated with the Department of Psychiatry, Novosibirsk Medical Institute.

The unitary stereotype concept presupposes the notion of equivalency in all forms of alcoholism. This basic concept leads to a convergence of thinking about alcohol which is not really new. Leonhard (1979), for example, noted that ". . . the theory of the 'unitary psychosis,' which was current more than a 100 years ago, has reappeared in new clothing." The issue thus becomes one of determining the implications of such thinking.

All variables involved in human drinking behavior, viewed from this disease perspective, are perceived as an expression of an invisible but existing pathological process, the so-called "pathogenesis of alcoholism" or "Pathos." Although no one has ever directly observed this "Pathos," or whatever it might be called — "bad habit," "payment for father's sins," "evil," and so on — everybody can thing about "Pathos" and its demonic destructive effects. Many pathways guide "Pathos" to a single nosology — "Alcoholism" — like the small rivers which flow into a big river, and the big rivers which then flow into the sea. This convergence represents a "mind-trap," and leads to generalizations which give us a false understanding of alcoholism which is expressed in words or terms such as "clinical case." This approach restricts intellectual curiosity from seeking new information. But if intellectual curiosity is "switched off," one's mind may fall into the trap of a closed theoretical system which exists as "special knowledge" in the individual's mind. An outline of "special narcological knowledge," based on a maximum convergent model of alcoholism, is represented in Figure 1. It has a pyramid's form and a strict hierarchy in its inner logical structure. The top of the pyramid is a high level of generalization of pure nosological thinking. It is a controlling part of the body of knowledge, where "Nosos" is pattern, which connects "Pathos" and its pathways into "thought system," called "clinical syndromes," which connects to other parts: biochemistry, pharmacology, physiology, psychology and so on. Within the hierarchy the lower level is supervised and controlled by the higher level of generalization. This clinical thinking is a kind of perceptive filter, which controls the process of information gathering, decision making and other mental processes utilized by specialists who treat alcoholics. Their treatment approach, however, has been conditioned by his or her "clinical vision."

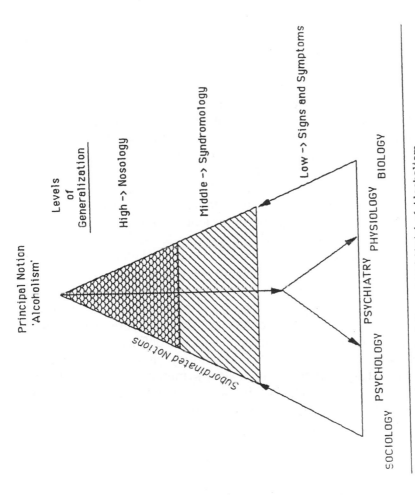

Figure 1. Convergent Model of Alcoholism

In this pyramid a secret formula (i.e., a presupposition) is hidden: If alcoholism exists then there must be alcoholics. Of course, alcoholism exists — it's an axiom. But what about alcoholics? Where are they? How are they detected? Who are they, i.e., what is an "alcoholic personality?" and so on. Formally, these questions might have been resolved by using clinical thinking, which gave the specialist a basis to respond to a clinical case.

Perhaps 200 years ago, before the disease concept of alcoholism was introduced, scientists used another approach: If alcoholics exist, then there must be alcoholism. Alcoholics were in existence because heavy drinking people always existed in real life — this was an axiom. But many years ago there was no "special knowledge" about alcoholism. Scientists, however, relied on the timeless process of formal logic in their approach to alcoholism — "If . . . then . . ." was created to connect the axioms, propositions, descriptions and explanations in the "thought systems," "pyramids," or complex tautology that were established to explain alcoholism.

Altschuler (1983) believes that all alcoholics have alcoholism (an axiom), but that alcoholism itself may have different forms. It is generally accepted by researchers and practitioners that there are different expressions of alcoholism. One of these variations is called the "obligatory syndrome," which is defined as a pathological craving for alcohol (PCA), which may involve paranoiac, obsessive, paroxysmal and hallucinatory symptoms ("Pathos" and its pathways). This is a clearly defined clinical picture which takes into account overt clinical symptoms. Altschuler, however, believes that all alcoholic patients that are not overtly psychotic or neurotic are "ordinary alcoholics" who nevertheless have invisible pathology. Altschuler's thinking is clearly contradictory, and represents a clinging to fixed ideas about alcoholism. Moreover, if a practitioner is locked into only detecting possible varieties of PCA, then it would be easy for him or her to choose the corresponding scheme of psychopharmacological correlation of alcoholic disease. This practice, however, works only when the clinician is confronted with a special form of alcoholism (i.e., PCA), but fails when applied to other possible manifestations.

Dealing with the complexities of the problem of alcohol dependence is simplified by a convergent manner of thinking. When a specialist has only one model of alcoholism to be concerned about, and only one way to describe and explain human problems, he/she appears to be in a very dangerous situation because they lose their flexibility and may thus encounter difficulty in relating to other human beings. This process is illustrated by the statement: "This man is an alcoholic, because I think he is." No doubt, convergence leads to an abstract construct, the so-called "ideal statistical alcoholic," whose "behavior" is predictable, understandable and compacted into well-subordinated notions of the pyramid.

In contrast to fixed ideas, a divergent approach does not concern itself with specific nosologies or with the classification of individuals, but accepts individuals as a unique holistic system, in which each person has their own picture of the world and their private "inner world." This pattern of thinking generates new, more vivid mental constructs, images and notions, more concrete terms and words, all of which are representative of an individual's behavior. There is no description of "pathways of Pathos," but "Individual Pathways." The models and information, used as "special knowledge," have no hierarchical structure (Velichokovsky, 1983). It means that theories, hypotheses and perspectives of any discipline are all equivalent, and therefore there is no "monopoly of truth" in any particular discipline. (Figure 2 presents a schematic of the divergent model.)

A new hypothesis about alcohol dependence must be created for every patient, that is, every case must be perceived as unique. An important question arises: Will the system work in psychotherapy, will it be useful for a specialist to help a patient change his or her behavior? The divergent approach is responsive to any form of alcoholism, even those cases which may involve tension reduction, latent homosexuality, dependence-independence conflict, or family disruption. But any diagnosis or understanding of a particular form of alcoholism does not necessarily apply to other cases. The results of group studies or statistical models, therefore, cannot be applied to an individual.

The divergent approach is analogous to a single-case method in medicine and in medical psychology (Yule & Hemsley, 1977), which involves an attempt to understand the unique problem of an individual, an attempt to describe some "psychological processes which may be at fault" (Yule & Hemsley, 1977, p. 212). Recog-

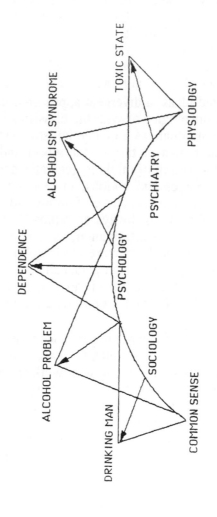

Figure 2. Divergent Model of Alcoholism.

nizing and changing these defective psychological processes, whatever they may be called—"alcohol problems," "psychological dependence," "addictive behavior," "craving for alcohol," "alcoholic games," and so on—is of paramount importance. "The map is not the territory, and the name is not the thing named" (Bateson, 1979, p. 32). We can not help patients by labeling them as alcoholic, and by only stressing a proper diagnosis based on clinical rules or schemes. But it is difficult for a patient to find treatment without a "diagnosis-ticket" (medical documents) to gain entry to treatment. It is also difficult for a therapist to justify his or her professional help without "diagnosis making."

Thus, there are two contrary manners of world viewing: (1) the convergent view, which perceives a world governed by laws (Pierce, 1976), and which advocates that only through the organization of information about reality is it possible to predict future events and to recognize their consequences, and (2) the divergent view, which helps us to recognize events with unpredictable consequences and which creates new realities that open potential possibilities about the meaning of life.

These two viewpoints, representing discrete and continuous types of thinking, respectively, are bipolar—"rigor verses imagination." As Bateson (1979) put it, there are ". . . rigor and imagination, the two great contraries of mental process, either of which by itself is lethal. Rigor alone is paralytic death, but imagination alone is insanity" (p. 242). An appropriate synchrony and harmony between rigor and imagination, between convergent and divergent manners of thinking, and between two theoretic-informative structures of knowledge, are the keystones of a new approach to alcoholism. The first attempt to utilize this approach, referred to as a "clinical-psychological analysis of alcoholism," was undertaken in Novosibirsk in the 1970s.

THE CLINICAL-PSYCHOLOGICAL APPROACH

The initial application of the clinical-psychological analysis of alcoholism, referred to as the Novosibirsk school of thought on alcoholism, grew out of a scientific study of alcoholism by Korolenko and Dickovsky (1971). These authors suggested a new classification of alcoholism which broke through the stereotypical thinking represented by the unitary concept of alcoholism. Their approach represented a synthesis of Jellinek's disease concept, particularly his classification of five distinct subtypes of alcohol abuse, and on his traditional clinical definitions of alcoholism. Their scheme is based on differences between two main aspects of the problem: (1) *The form*, i.e., forms of "alcohol dependence syndrome," representing formation process of all the variants of alcohol addiction; and (2) *The stage*, i.e., stages of "psycho-organic syndrome," representing the dynamics of exogenous-organic brain disturbances as a process caused by the direct impact of alcohol on the central nervous system.

Both types — "form" and "stage" — leave sufficient room for seeing phenomenon in a broad perspective. The first one defines alcoholism in terms of psychological-socio-cultural dimensions rather than in clinical terms. The second perspective approaches alcoholism in terms of classical psychiatry and neurology. Theoretically, the term "form" can be used to refer to numerous variables involved in the alcohol dependence syndrome, and is closely related to Pattison's "multivariate model of alcoholism syndrome" (Pattison, 1979). Korolenko's classification scheme includes nine forms of alcoholism: *Alpha, Eta, Iota, Kappa*, within which "psychological dependence" predominate, and *Gamma, Delta, Zeta, Theta*, and *Epsilon*, within which "physical dependence" on alcohol predominate. These classifications are open ended and may vary to account for new forms of alcoholism.

The concept of "stage" can be used to describe the many different kind of signs and symptoms of mental disorders and psychiatric problems found in alcoholics, ranging from slight deterioration of mental functions ("cerebrastenia" stage), to more severe mental problems, including memory deficit, cognitive, affective and personality disturbances, psychotic transitory symptoms ("encephalopathy" stage), to hard mental disorders, including "intellectual degradation," "severe personality changes," chronic states of acoustic hallucination or paranoiac ideas, and other psychopathological symptoms ("partial dementia" stage). There are certain correlations between different forms of the alcohol dependence syndrome and stages of the psycho-organic brain syndrome, but this classification scheme is sufficiently flexible to describe the alcohol problem in detail (Korolenko, 1978; Korolenko & Timofejeva, 1986). This approach is not unlike the concern with the issue of dual diagnosis currently emerging in the United States.

Research has tended to support the stage and form types of alcoholism. For example, while analyzing two types of alcoholism — alpha and eta — a "motivational model" was suggested by Zavjalov (1981). According to this model psychological dependence on alcohol is a concept, denoting sets of specific psychological phenomena associated with a given person's alcohol problem, which involves the following: (1) an expectation of positive effects from drinking, which establishes, no matter how one imagines it, false beliefs, attitudes, or myths about how alcohol will help one to feel better, (2) motives for drinking behavior, and (3) ritual drinking, habitual drinking, group drinking, or other socially acquired, learned behavior patterns, all manifested in an appropriate social context of drinking. All three of these can serve as possible means for alcoholics to justify their drinking.

The ongoing psychological processes — expectancy, motives and rituals — interact with each other and result in a complex condition. Serving as the "core" of a person's alcohol problem, this complex condition is transformed into specific symptoms that the clinician may describe as a special syndrome or as an uncertain set of symptoms. The condition can be properly diagnosed by a careful observer who is in close personal contact with the patient. This complex condition is referred to as personal reasons for drinking (Zavjalov, 1988).

It must be emphasized that in a specific sociocultural context, and in certain environments, the Clinical-Psychological model leads to a conceptualization of "multiple versions" of alcohol dependence, which require different therapeutic strategies. The Clinical-Psychological model has been described more fully in two recent publications: "Personality and Alcohol" (Korolenko & Zavjalov, 1987), and "Psychological Aspects of Alcohol Dependence Formation" (Zavjalov, 1988). The main statements of this approach are summarized below.

1. The phenomenon that is described and explained using the terms alcoholism, alcohol dependence, problem drinking, etc., can be studied from two different viewpoints, and it is possible to arrive

at two different descriptions of the problem studied — a clinical description and a psychological description. Each of these descriptions provides useful information about drinking behavior. This information can be helpful in gathering, classifying and assessing information that is needed to help a patient to change his or her behavior.

2. The very essence of "disease" or "psychological state" of a person with an alcohol problem can be revealed only by personal contact through appropriate communication with the patient in the therapist-patient-context interaction. The clinician must obtain a personality profile and a history of the drinking behavior. If the clinician is only interested in asking how, where, when, and with whom a person drinks, there is insufficient knowledge to adequately understand the patient's problems. When this occurs the patient is treated as an object, isolated from his or her national culture, ethnicity, symbols and personal values, micro and macrosocial milieu, his or her own world view, and self-awareness. The results lead to a limited abstract scheme or "alcoholic image" which may misguide the therapist. Careful attention should be given to:

a. The patient's world view (PWV), which is a reflection of his or her personal ideology and thought system, convictions and ideas, including one's inner picture of the disease, and everything that characterizes him or her.
b. The therapist's world view (TWV), which represents the therapist's personal orientation regarding psychological processes, signs of disease, and learned technical skills.

The interaction of both these phenomena results in a clearer diagnosis and facilitates a dialogue between the therapist and client, even though each of them maintain different subjective experiences and fulfill different roles. Emphasis is not on diagnosis, which can result in treating the patient as a label, but is placed instead on a process of constantly gathering information to understanding the client.

3. Psychotherapy is understood as a process of dialogue between a therapist and a patient, involving an exchange of their world

views. Specific psychological problems, inappropriate behaviors, problems of interacting with social organizations, and difficulties in interpersonal relations, among other problems, are discussed with the aim of arriving at a solution.

The interaction between the therapist and patient represents a microcosm of the way the patient acts in the real world. A joint effort is undertaken to find ways of recognizing and solving the patient's problems. The therapist, however, doesn't actually solve a patient's problems, but only helps him/her to learn how to solve them. Psychotherapy is thus "learning to learn" through imagination, metacognition, "mental experiments" and "remodeling" of the ongoing psychological processes of past and future events.

4. An appropriate understanding of the psychotherapeutic process occurs when it is perceived as a dialogue, involving an interrelationship, the main function of which is the realization and reconstruction of the client's conceptual model of the world. It means that the therapist needs to be aware of how relative any conceptual model may be as it applies to the client, no matter what indisputable authority espouses it. The clinician has to be able to modify his or her conceptual models in order to match the client's needs if an effective intervention is to be achieved. Ideally, the therapist is a skilled person who is a "universal communicator" — a man or woman with convictions and idea systems — who is open to new views, can accept different conceptual models and revise them to be useful for each individual.

Failure to consider the client's perspective can result in "clinical dogmatism," in which the therapist imposes his/her own clinical model instead of understanding the client's world view. For example, telling a client directly that he/she has a "pathological craving for alcohol," does not help the patient to understand the nature of the problem. Just helping the client to identify the problem without understanding it in context of its etiology, its proper definition, or effects on behavior, can result in the client resisting the problem rather than to begin to deal with it.

5. The Clinical-Psychological approach allows us to synthesize thinking from different scientific disciplines, to study alcohol problems with versatility in mind, and to go beyond the limits of partiality to a particular model of alcoholism. In brief, a multivariate ap-

proach, which encompasses neurological, psychiatric and psychological aspects, is more apt to work with clients who seek help. Furthermore, the multivariate approach used in psychotherapy helps the therapist to be more human and to think independently.

TOWARDS A NEW PSYCHOTHERAPEUTIC METHODOLOGY

The Clinical-Psychological approach to alcoholism provides a different frame of reference when compared to traditional thinking, one which encourages the therapist to think independently in response to the client's needs. Independence is defined as becoming free from rigid medical models, to recognize the limitations of labeling alcoholism as a disease — in the narrow sense of the word — and to also recognize limitations of treatment approaches which only focus on symptom reduction. As Suarex and Mills (1983) wrote: "True psychological principles are not amenable to personal 'use,' in the sense that they could be used on people, or by people in a manipulative way on one another. They are 'impersonal' in the sense that they are like the principles of mathematics, they impersonally describe the results of certain key relationships between our thought, our experiences and our behavior . . ." (p. 29).

In treating people with alcohol-related problems, the process of psychotherapy is focussed on the Patient's World View (PWV) and the ways of changing it. Psychotherapy is an integral part of the alcoholism treatment program and has its own levels of therapeutic intervention, which range from short-term psychotherapy, which involves a very intensive intervention focussed on the patient's current problems, to long-term psychotherapy, which involves well-planned, systematic, educative interventions ". . . directed toward specific targets of psychic change in specific alcoholics (Pattison, 1979, p. 157).

CHANGING PERSONAL MOTIVES

Zavjalov (1988), following a series of studies of alcohol consumption, identified motivation as the key problem in psychological dependence and *Motives of Alcohol Consumption* (MAC) were defined as a precise and concrete target of therapeutic intervention.

The term motivation refers to a very complex psychobiological cycle of behavior found in people dependent on alcohol: need → want → seek → take → dependence → withdraw → need → . Alcohol motivation is closely connected with alcohol adaptation. On a psychological level, certain types of alcohol consumption motivation can be differentiated through psychological testing and through clinical interviews. Nine *psychosemantic* types were described in the MAC model:

1. Traditional (customs, feasts, "special cases," etc.).
2. Submissive ("alcoholic pressure," forced conjoint drinking, etc.).
3. Pseudo-cultural (drinking alcohol as a status symbol, cultural drinking, imitation, etc.).
4. Hedonistic (psychosomatic pleasure, "high" mood, etc.).
5. Ataractic (drinking to reduce anxiety or fears).
6. Hyperactive or stimulative (sensation-seeking, overcoming, avoiding, etc.).
7. Medical (self-medicating, overcoming withdrawal symptoms or other health problems).
8. Addictive (altering consciousness, addictive behavior, etc.).
9. Protest and self-destructive motivation.

Thus the psychological content of alcohol dependence is represented as a certain combination of these types or predominance of one of them (Zavjalov, 1988).

Several therapeutic approaches — question-response techniques, interpretation, persuasion, reframing and reflecting — are helpful in psychotherapy for these types of motivation to be "talked out" as personal themes. Therapy is aimed at changing a patient's rigid mental schemes. The process involves dealing with the semantic structure of psychological content and to encourage the patient to talk freely.

It is possible to examine some explicit definitions of motivation which could be used in psychotherapy. While working out our own method of MAC exploration, we carefully sorted verbal expressions of alcohol experience and causal explanations. In such a way an explicit definition of motive can be defined as a *linear verbal code* to represent personal patterns which connects cause and effect. For example, in Siberia, a usual reason to drink is expressed as "I drink after hard work." The patient gives us a verbal message about the way he used to connect "drink" (event Y or effect) with hard work (event X or cause). The important word here is *after*, because in the patient's own mind the original statement "I drink after hard work" can be modified into "I drink because I'm hard working" — connecting two real independent events — drink and work — in a cause-effect semantic group. Treatment then has to focus on breaking the patient's self-established perception of the relationship between work and drinking.

The patient may also describe his or her personal views to the therapist, telling stories about his/her own drinking problem, but in fact may be talking about how other people drink, or about friends' drinking behavior. Sometimes the patient can describe his own alcohol experience indirectly, telling the therapist some kind of legend, fable, tale, or anecdotes describing absurd situations. Such stories are often called *alcoholic alibis* and are classified as symptoms of moral degradation by some clinical psychiatrists. However, we assume that they may be taken as a legitimate target for psychotherapeutic intervention through imagery techniques (Shorr, 1983). The assumption is that these alcoholic alibis represent an incorporation of society's views about drinking. Imagery techniques help the patient to differentiate between his or her own personal values and those held by society as a whole. The aim of this process is to help the client to identify and deal with his or her own problem in terms of what meaning it has to him or her.

SUMMARY

A Clinical-Psychological approach has been briefly outlined. This approach is proposed as just one of many methods which can be used in the treatment of patients with alcohol-related problems. The Clinical-Psychological approach does not represent a simple combination of clinical and psychological thinking, but represents instead a new methodology to study, explain, and treat alcohol-related problems. This clinical system is based on the belief that the client is not only the object of study but is also an active participant whose views are to be taken into consideration. The procedure is believed to help facilitate a broader perspective and deeper understanding of the patient's inner world that is related to his/her drinking behavior.

LIST OF REFERENCES

Altschuler, V.B. (1983) Correlation between main syndrome of chronic alcoholism. *Journal of Neuropathology and Psychiatry*, *4*, 596-600.

Bateson, F. (1979). *Mind and nature: A necessary unity*. NY: Bantam Books.

Bekhtel, E. Ye. (1986). *Prenosological forms of alcohol abuse*. Moscow: Meditsina.

Korolenko, C.P. (1978). *The psychophysiological adaptation in extreme conditions*. Leningrad: Meditsina.

Korolenko, C.P., & Dickovsky, A.A. (1971). Clinical variants of alcoholism. In C.P. Korolenko (Ed.), *Problems of clinical and experimental psychiatry* (pp. 3-8).

Korolenko, C.P., & Timofejeva, A.S. (1986). *The Roots of Alcoholism*. Novosibirsk, USSR.

Korolenko, C.P., & Zavjalov, V. Yu. (1987). *Personality and Alcohol*. Novosibirsk, USSR: "Nauka" (Science-Press).

Pattison, M.E. (1979). The selection of treatment modalities for the alcoholic patient. In J.H. Mendelson & N.K. Mello (Eds.), *The Diagnosis and Treatment of Alcoholism* (pp. 125-228). NY: McGraw-Hill.

Shorr, J.E. (1983). *Psychotherapy through imagery* (2nd ed). NY: Time-Stratton Inc.

Suarez, E.M., & Mills, R.C. (1983). *Sanity, insanity and common sense: The missing link in understanding mental health*. Aurora, Illinois: Med.-Psych. Publications.

Velichkovsky, B.A., & Kapitsa, M.S. (1987). The psychological problems of intellect study. In E.P. Velikhov (Ed.), *Intellectual processes and their modeling* (pp. 120-141). Moscow: Nauka (Science Press).

Yule, W., & Hemsley, D. (1977). Single-case method in medical psychology. In S. Rachman (Ed.), *Contributions to Medical Psychology. Vol. 1* (pp. 211-229). NY: Pergamon Press.

Zavjalov, V. Yu. (1988) *Psychological aspects of alcohol dependence formation*. Novosibirsk, USSR: "Nauka" (Science Press).

Social-Psychological Aspects of Drinking by Youth and Young Adults

A. S. Timofeeva, MD
L. F. Perekrjostova, MD

During recent years the growth and distribution of alcoholism in many countries of the world has resulted in a large number of studies devoted to the problem of alcohol use by young people. This is a particularly interesting and challenging problem for us because we have found that early abuse of alcohol tends, as a rule, to be the basis for establishing a progressive course of abusive drinking, and leads to a rapid onset of personality change together with a loss of social contacts and a change in associated behaviors.

Most investigations have focused on either an analysis of traits formed in early childhood or on teenage alcoholism, or tend to study the influence of early alcohol use on the dynamics of personality change. Another area of interest has been on studying the onset of drinking behavior among young criminals (Lichko, 1977; Gurjeva & Gindikin, 1980; Makarov, 1981; Artemchuk, 1985).

There are only a few studies in Soviet research which have investigated drinking patterns among healthy, non-problem-drinking teenagers, or which have examined the social and psychological factors linked to early alcohol use by young people (Tedder & Sidorov, 1976; Lisitsin & Kopyt, 1983). Tedder and Sidorov, who studied the context and amount of alcohol consumed by youth, found that 49.8% of the boys and 31.0% of the girls drank alcohol at least once by the age of 16 or 17. These authors concluded that drinking among youth starts at the age of 10 or 11 for girls, and at the age of nine for boys. They concluded that there is a need to

A. S. Timofeeva and L. F. Perekrjostova are affiliated with the Department of Psychiatry, Novosibirsk Medical Institute.

begin to teach children about alcohol during the first stages of elementary school, and that if prevention efforts are to be effective it is essential to know how early drinking behavior starts and under what circumstances it develops.

Our investigations have shown a high prevalence of drinking alcohol at an early age, and alcohol problems among groups of healthy teenagers and among teenagers who manifest antisocial and criminal behavior. We identified four developmental stages which are related to teenage alcoholism.

1. Adaptation to Alcohol

This stage begins with the first experience with alcohol, usually between the ages of 7 and 11. The first experience with alcohol occurs in the family or with older schoolmates. This first taste of alcohol is usually experienced as unpleasant, largely because of its burning sensation and unpleasant after-effects. Drinking is seldom repeated after this early initiation. Most young children do not want to drink, but those who continue do so out of submission to the influence of older teenagers who themselves tend to drink. At this time they become acquainted with the effect of different alcoholic beverages, and begin to define their ability to handle alcohol. After drinking most children experience unpleasant feelings, but others experience feelings of pleasure. However, they seldom tell about experiencing a good mood during intoxication because they did not begin to achieve a sense of euphoria. The most frequent motives given for drinking are to experience new feelings, to associate with grown-ups, to act as grown-ups and to assert their independence.

Adequate educative and pedagogical measures at this stage can stop youthful drinking, but if the drinking proceeds the second stage begins at about 2-3 months following their initiation to drinking.

2. Confirmation of Stereotypes of Alcohol Behavior

During this period an active tendency to use alcohol develops. Youngsters become deeply acquainted with different alcoholic beverages, and find the best type for themselves. At this stage they begin to learn that alcohol improves mood, but alcohol effects each youngster differently. Some feel relaxation, others experience an increase in activity and become more aggressive. These two reactions become the motive which is expressed most often for using hard liquor or wine. At this stage any previous unpleasant experience with alcoholic beverages begins to dissipate.

Most important, is that during this stage the young drinkers begin to attempt to control their drinking to obtain a mild level of intoxication. But this attempt does not prevent severe intoxication. Any relationships with nondrinking friends begins to weaken. Contacts with older, drinking teenagers are strengthened. Teenagers attempt to cover up their intoxication from grown-ups through flaunting one another. Alcohol excess is reinforced by the group members themselves, the presence of alcohol in the family, access to money, and a lot of free time. The reasons most often given for drinking are: to improve mood, to kill time, to escape from reality, to relax, and to increase self-confidence. These motives are also related to the drinking that occurs during the first stage.

The second stage does not represent any form of alcoholism because there is no dependence on alcohol, and drinking can be stopped by pedagogical and educative measures. If drinking does not stop the transition to the next stage occurs between 2 months to a year after the second stage is firmly established.

3. Psychological Dependence on Alcohol

The first real alcohol-related problem behavior or symptoms of alcoholism begin with the establishment of psychological dependence. The youthful drinkers are no longer children, but are beginning to enter their teens, and are no longer influenced by the actions of older-drinking adolescents. They have become active drinkers and drink without encouragement from others. They are usually aware of all known alcoholic beverages and their substitutes. There is an inclination for alcohol not only in the evening but in the daytime as well. Alcohol intoxication becomes the most desirable psychic state. Everything begins to change as a result of drinking. Studying, family, sports and hobbies become unimportant. Achievement in school suffers greatly. With the development of psychological dependence on alcohol the behavior of teenagers is defined by their desire to drink alcohol. They lose contacts with members of their former groups and find new friends. They use all their free time to look for alcohol and speak only about drinking; they also entertain and solve their conflicts only in an intoxicated state. Sometimes, by staying in their former group, they provoke friends to use alcohol. Such teenagers have no sense of responsibility connected with family, school, or social problems because all of their interests are both directly and indirectly associated with alcohol.

Drinking tends to improve their mood. An attempt is made to mask drinking through group behavior. Free time spent without alcohol is defined as dull, as time without entertainment. At such times the possibility to commit some type of criminal act is high.

The most typical motives for drinking in this stage are: a tendency to be part of the group, a desire to be intoxicated, to improve mood, and to feel grown-up.

This stage lasts from several months to a year and a half. Not only pedagogical and educative measures but medical help is also necessary if an effective intervention is to be made.

4. Physical Dependence on Alcohol

The most important symptoms of this stage of physical dependence are: seeking the euphoria involved with intoxication, loss of control, inability to abstain, and the onset of withdrawal symptoms. At this stage physical dependence on alcohol is not only maintained, but also increases. Tolerance to alcohol is greatly increased (4-5 times compared with the beginning), and the vomiting reflex is usually lost. Many teenagers prefer strong alcoholic drinks. If they have neither wine nor vodka they can drink different substitutes in order to satisfy their need. When the syndrome of loss of control is developed even small doses of alcohol can induce a desire to drink more. As a rule, each drinking episode results in a state of deep intoxication. Sometimes intoxication with amnesia occurs.

The alcohol syndrome among teenagers, however, is not always clearly defined. Oftentimes, teenagers feel guilty after excessive drinking, which may be important because guilt is considered to be a one of the classic symptoms of alcoholic behavior. An inclination to drink first thing in the morning also indicates that withdrawal symptoms may be beginning to appear. Such teenagers also show symptoms which are consistent with adult symptoms, such as mood change, depression, self-depreciation, increased irritation, horrible dreams and nightmares.

At this stage the motives to use alcohol are closely related to the motives that exist during the first stage: a tendency to be close to grown-ups, to change feelings, to feel self-important, etc. As we observe the process of teenage alcoholism develop, we have found that reasons for drinking depend not only on the personality traits of a teenager, but also to a great extent on the conditions of education. Teenage alcohol abusers try to choose friends who also drink, and induce other teenagers to join them. Children with an unhappy family life, or who come from homes with emotional instability, or who are in conflict with their parents, or who come from homes where parents reject them, are especially vulnerable to drink in a group. Such teenagers begin to prefer street friends to family. There is an increasing tendency to substitute peer support for parental support. Parental control decreases, and parental authority diminishes, misunderstanding and estrangement intensifies. We have found that when such conditions arise the children perceive themselves as unwanted or unnecessary. They are sad, depressed, and indifferent about their appearance. They often hide their depressed mood by expressing undue familiarity, telling rough jokes, and acting aggressively. Alcohol assists in maintaining a roughness and aggressiveness, which results in further estrangement and isolation from the family.

It should be noted that such teenagers reveal contrasting symptoms during the early and late periods of their consistent drinking. The earliest syndrome presents a series of symptoms which consist of heightened levels of irritation, anger and aggressiveness. Such adolescents express undue familiarity and cynicism, and they become severe egotists. Emotional dulling takes place. One's sphere of interests becomes very narrow and they lose interest in life events, and seek to escape from their homes. Intellectual activity decreases and they often give up studying or work.

Another clinical picture consists of psychic instability and easy suggestibility. Simultaneously, there is a general tone of mood change. We can see carelessness and light-mindedness in some cases, anger and indifference, especially toward parents. A higher level of suggestibility and impulsiveness (especially in an alcoholic state), together with undeveloped social-moral values (a feeling of duty, responsibility), lead such teenagers to commit crimes. According to Gurjeva and Gindikin (1980), the number of young criminals who are problem drinkers range from 14.3 to 31.6 percent, while the number suffering from alcoholism ranges from 5.2 to 26.2 percent. Our research has shown that among adolescents who committed criminal acts and who were referred for a clinical evaluation, 25 percent were psychologically dependent on alcohol, and 9.7 percent were physically dependent.

In summary, our discussion points toward the need for teachers and clinical practitioners to identify children at high risk for development of alcohol-related problems as early as possible. Among those at high risk, one of the most important contributing factors is coming from an unhappy family relationship. Teenagers who consistently act tough or aggressively and who are involved in criminal acts are also at high risk.

It is especially important to take note of which teenagers drink together, and to attempt to change the group's attitudes and values. Helping these youngsters to learn how to deal more effectively with their problems may help to reduce, if not eliminate, their drinking behavior. They must be patiently educated to develop proper attitudes toward alcohol. It should be noted that prevention of early alcoholism must be tied to broad governmental social actions encouraging healthy lifestyles.

LIST OF REFERENCES

Artemchuk, A.F. (1985). *Alcoholism in youth*. Kiev: Zdorovja.

Gurjeva, V.A., & Gindinkin, V. Ja. (1980). *Psychopathy and alcoholism in youth*. Moscow.

Korolenko, C.P. & Timofeeva, A.S. (1986). *The roots of alcoholism*. Novosibirsk.

Lichko, A.E. (1977). *Psychopathies and accentuations of character in teenagers*. Leningrad: Meditsina.

Makarov, V.V. (1981). Alcoholism development in teenagers. *Autoref. Diss. Cand. Medical Science*. Novosibirsk.

Tedder, Ju. P., & Sidorov, P.I. (1976). Particular socio-hygenic aspects of alcohol habits development. *Sovjetskoje Zdravoochranenie*, 4.

Lisitsin, Ju. P. & Kopyt, N. Ya. (1983). *Alcoholism (socio-hygenic aspects)*. Moscow: Meditsina.

Addictive Behavior in Women:
A Theoretical Perspective

C. P. Korolenko, MD
T. A. Donskih, MD

THEORETICAL PERSPECTIVE

The analysis of events which take place in a society, such as deviant behavior (behavior that is considered to border on or depart from socially acceptable ethics and morals), leads to observations and conclusions about the event, which then tends to bring about an increase in the behavior studied. These increased deviations are discovered in various fields of contemporary life and have diverse manifestations. Belonging in this category, for example, are such behaviors as stealing, violent crimes, aggressive behavior among certain groups of people, such as fanatics, black marketers and corrupters, gambling, and the misuse of various substances for the purpose of achieving an altered state of consciousness. The variety of these deviant behaviors leads to a situation in which such disorders come under the care of different medical specialists and different disciplines, which include medicine, education, police, social workers, etc. The necessity for such a diverse effort is brought about by the specific features of the different disorders. However outwardly different these deviations may appear, they nevertheless have some specific common characteristics. Discovery of these common characteristics may be significant for prevention and treatment of these problems.

Essential to establishing a common understanding of these different behavioral manifestations is the derivation of a term that unites

C. P. Korolenko and T. A. Donskih are affiliated with the Novosibirsk Medical Institute.

them. The term *deviance* has recently been cited by researchers, especially in sociological literature. In a sociological context, the investigation of deviant behavior reflects the nature of social problems and the level of tension in a society.

One form of deviant behavior is *addictive behavior*. Addictive behavior may be defined as a desire to escape from reality by means of changing one's mental state, usually achieved by using substances with narcotic effects, including alcohol. Such an alteration of consciousness, however, is not limited to using drugs. Prolonged listening to rhythmically accentuated music, for example, or psychological exercises (meditation, yoga), can also induce an altered state of consciousness to help an individual escape from reality. Other forms of addictive behavior involve gambling or eating, either of which is qualitatively and quantitatively different from drug use or self-induced psychological change. As such, alcoholism and other forms of drug abuse both represent different forms of the overall problem of addictive behavior, which itself is a representation of the much broader problem of deviant behavior.

Alcohol and drugs are not new to societies in most parts of the world. The current history in the USSR, however, is marked by a new dimension of addictive behavior—the widespread use of alcohol as well as many different kinds of mind-altering substances by large segments of society. A similar situation has also been described with respect to drug use in the United States (Segal, 1988).

The use of the term addictive behavior is very operative. It may reveal the peculiarities of the development of alcoholism, narcotic addiction, and forms of drug addiction, each of which has been considered to be a separate entity by specialists in addiction studies. When each of these problems are treated separately (i.e., a narrow approach), rather than as different manifestations of an addictive disorder, there is a strong risk of making not only a tactical error but also a strategic error, either of which, over time, can be costly. The narrow view contributes to create a public and professional attitude that calls for "the eradication of evil," (i.e., attacks against drinking). These attacks are based on an over-simplified explanation of alcoholism, which relies on an eclectic combination of formal logic, pseudo-emotional fervor, and an appeal to common sense.

This is especially dangerous when such programs are created as a result of group pressure from people who are fanatically convinced that all forms of addiction are unrelated phenomena and are responsive to some rather simple form of treatment.

A recent and very illustrative example of such a situation was the attempt to solve the alcohol problem in the USSR with the help of predominantly prohibition-like measures affecting the production and sale of alcohol. It was possible to predict that there would be some negative consequences of such action based on the experience of attempts at prohibition in other countries during the 20th century, such as Iceland, Norway, the United States (1920-1932), Russia and the USSR (1914-1925), and Poland (1981 to 1983). Some of the negative consequences that were recorded in these countries were an increase in home-brewing, black market profiteering, the appearance of organized criminality associated with illegal production and sale of alcohol, and an increase in intoxication through various types of substances which change one's mental state. Although these results varied in each country, the nature of their variation was strongly dependent on local social and cultural factors. For example, in the United States, the development of organized criminal gangs such as the mafia was an important byproduct of Prohibition. In Russia and the USSR, production of home-brewed brandy increased. In Poland production of home distilled alcohols, black marketing, decrease in sugar supplies, and an increase in intoxication through the use of other drugs and various toxic substances were noted.

Korolenko and Timofeeva (1986) attempted to report that prohibition-like efforts would not be totally effective but, unfortunately, their opinions were not in conformance with popular opinion, and were not taken into consideration. More recently, however, recognition has been paid to the realization that the attempt to limit alcohol has not been successful in eliminating alcohol-related problems. Additionally, there is an increasing awareness that addictive behavior has many different manifestations, and that these behaviors differ from what has been traditionally defined as classical addiction.

The concept of classical addiction is nevertheless repeatedly quoted in Soviet psychiatric textbooks. But the clinical picture regarding narcotic addiction has changed so dramatically in the USSR that today's cases no longer match the classical description. Thus the description of the classical narcotic addict is no longer relevant. In other words, psychiatric thinking has failed to keep up with changes in the field.

It must be stressed that there is a need to move from the old position of classical addiction to the more modern concept of addictive disorders. The concept of addictive disorders is currently utilized in our clinic in Novosibirsk, and is part of our theoretical scheme that explains the development of addiction from its inception. Within the context of this framework, for example, narcotic addiction is seen as beginning as a primary desire to take narcotic substances with the aim of inducing a change of one's mental state largely out of curiosity, or as a search for new and exciting sensations. In the case of classical narcotic addictions, the development of the process begins differently — narcotics are first taken as a result of a doctor's prescription to treat pain, but repeated use results in the development of psychological and physical dependence. This process has been referred to as pharmacologically-based addiction.

Contemporarily, this approach does not account for all the different forms of drug dependence that occur. Even when opiates are used, they are used primarily to change one's mood, to experience unusual sensations, to achieve psychological relaxation, and to induce a dream-like state. In addition to using drugs that have an analgesic effect to cause a change in consciousness, many other substances can be used such as various organic solvents or chemically modified drugs. When the substance of choice is unavailable the user seeks to substitute other drugs, but such changes only take place in the absence of strong physical dependency to the basic drug. Many substances do not induce physical dependence at all, but may contribute to severe organic disorders or brain damage with such clinical symptoms as memory loss, impoverishment of thinking, and a decrease in intellectual abilities.

We pay special attention to these peculiarities because effective preventive measures can not be based only on prohibition. Prohibition, when it is carried to an extreme to where it even bans over-the-counter medicines containing alcohol, is unduly restrictive for people who have no alcohol problems and who show little risk for development of alcohol dependence. People with addictive behavior are less affected from such limitations because they strive to find substitutes or turn to alternative drugs. A severe anti-addictive or prohibitive public policy is usually associated with a failure to understand the integral nature of the problem, which represents a complex interaction of many different factors. It must also be noted that the prohibition-like reaction to alcohol problems was not accidental. It resulted from an integration of attitudes about alcohol that prevailed in other fields such as sociology, economics, culture and education.

The discussion that follows applies some of the thinking expressed above to the study of addictive behavior in women. The results of the research presented is derived from an ongoing series of studies involving the principle authors and other clinical practitioners involved with the problem of addictive disorders in the Novosibirsk Medical Institute.

WOMEN AND ALCOHOL: THE RELATIONSHIP BETWEEN THEORY AND CLINICAL OBSERVATIONS

In the last decade more and more women have become involved in addictive behaviors. Their misuse of alcohol has become one of the most widespread problems in the USSR. The number of women drinking has doubled over the last ten years. In the 1970s in the USSR the number of women who drank was estimated to be approximately 5 percent[1] of the alcohol abusing population. It is now estimated to be about 10 percent.

An analysis of the characteristics of women alcoholics by us showed that among those who drank alcoholically, a large number first showed some form of deviant behavior that proceeded the development of alcohol dependence. This finding was most consistent among youth and young adult women who, before their drinking problems started, showed social problems, consistently violated ethical and cultural norms, and who had numerous sexual relations with casual partners. Many of these women who gravitated towards

---

1. All figures have been rounded to the nearest whole number.

criminal behavior did not have very strong attachment to their parents, relatives and friends. Their actions were based on a strong need to achieve immediate gratification without taking any consequences into consideration, even though intellectual ability was generally high. Once drinking started, the effects of drinking brought about a change in their motivation to drink. They now drank out of a desire to maintain a sense of stimulation, to alter impressions of reality, and to alter consciousness. As a whole, these women did not experience a deep emotional trauma in their lives or express feelings of shame and repentance. When confronted with their problems they always promised to improve, to "begin a new life," but they maintained their old ways. They are, however, able to make a positive impression, and even evoke sympathy and trust from people unacquainted with them.

One of the features of these alcoholic women consisted of an inability to endure loneliness, they do not like to be alone even for short periods of time. If they must be at home with parents or relatives for some reason, they listen to loud rhythmic music or talk over the telephone with their friends, who show the same behavior. They usually tend not to drink alone, but among others. They seek to obtain the alcohol's kef [dreamy condition] effect, and in some cases other substances are used in combination with alcohol or independently.

The character and the frequency of drinking and other drug use are connected with the characteristics of the group in which social relationships take place. Many women who act out are generally associated with other members of a group who also show antisocial tendencies. The types of social interaction and behavior are different for various groups, and there are variations of group dynamics. The forms of addictive behavior also vary. These women present a high risk for development of alcohol and drug dependency, sexually transmitted diseases, and are apt to commit criminal offenses.

Thus it can be clearly seen that there is an integral relationship between alcoholism, addictive behavior, and deviant behavior, and that treatment and prevention must proceed on a multidimensional level. For example, even if the drinking behavior is stopped, other problems remain, such as having to respond to periodic use of other drugs. In all these cases addictive behavior only changes its form of expression. A positive outcome can be obtained *only through the elimination of the motives contributing to the deviant behavior, and not by only treating some form of an addictive disorder.*

In context of learning more about the problem of women and alcohol, we investigated 160 women and teenage girls who ranged in age from 15 to 60 years old, all manifesting some form of deviant and addictive disorder. The sample group consisted of 20 schoolgirls, 35 college students, and a combination of 45 women who held skilled, unskilled and professional jobs, and 60 women who were unemployed. Extremely detailed psychiatric histories were obtained about their childhood and upbringing, and extensive psychological testing was also conducted (e.g., MMPI, Rorschach). Based on the results of this evaluation it was possible to identify some specific types of childhood rearing patterns that were found to be related to their deviant and addictive disorders. Six types of childhood experiences were derived.

Clinical Subgroups Based on Childhood Experiences

1. The first clinical subgroup, representing 33 percent of the cases, were all found to have clearly identifiable unfavorable childhood conditions. This was expressed by their having described a lack of parental attention, warmth, and emotional attachment. Many women (13%) came from single-parent homes, having been reared only by their mothers. Others came from a home situation involving a mother and stepfather, characterized by frequent quarrels, rows, and constant conflict between the girls and their stepfathers. From time to time these situations lead to serious fights which resulted in the girls running away. The parents were not interested in how their daughters succeeded at school and did not know how confused and troubled the girls were. The children felt lonely. They were often unsupervised by their parents. In many cases only bear necessities of food and clothing were provided — no emotional support was given. The girls did not have a positive image of their parents, and an emotional attachment to the home was absent. They did not like to return to their home, or to stay at home for long periods of time.

2. The second group (18% of the women) was composed of women who were brought up in an environment in which the families expressed antisocial attitudes. Of these women, 68% came from single-parent homes, with only the mother present. The mother's antisocial attitudes were expressed by frequent alcohol misuse, a lack of interest in meeting parental responsibilities, and sexual promiscuity. There was little parental emphasis on spiritual and intellectual development because they themselves showed little interest in these matters. The situation at home was one of child neglect, unsanitary conditions and, in many cases, the home represented nothing more than some type of night shelter to the child. The girls were constant witnesses to drinking-bouts, bawdy talk, fights, and to explicit sexual behavior by their mothers or fathers with casual sexual partners. In families without fathers, the father was usually in prison for thievery or hooliganism.

3. The third group (9% of the cases) was represented by women whose childhood was experienced in orphanages or boarding-schools. In all cases the children reared in orphanages were raised under extremely strict conditions. The staff and teachers did not establish any emotional relations with the children, which seemed to have instilled an avoidance in establishing close personal ties with people in general. These girls only anticipated trouble, humiliation and punishment from the staff. One significant factor was that it was practically impossible for the girls to be alone — there was always a steady presence of other children. The collective group of children created microgroups, each of which chose their own leaders and arranged their own rules, and any violations resulted in an immediate penalty. Great importance was attached to physical strength, to the ability to achieve something by deceiving adults, and by a display of independence. Their sexual interests began early. The girls who rose to leadership positions within the groups were seen as authority figures by the others, and they symbolized maturity and independence. In keeping with their roles, the leaders acted in an off-hand manner, smoked, flirted with boys, and drank alcohol, showing an unusual ability to consume large amounts but not to get drunk.

Each group's behavior reflected the personality of its leader. For example, if a leader was prone to juvenile delinquency the members of the group soon followed. The same pattern was observed with respect to the leader's drinking or use of other drugs.

4. The fourth group (21% of the cases) represented women who came from well-established upward mobile families who were striving to move ahead socially and economically. The girls were expected to be well dressed, their parents bought them fashionable clothes, and they were expected to conform to parental expectations. Significant attention was paid to the demonstration of an outward appearance of prosperity. The tendency to raise the prestige of the family was strongly accentuated. The parents were very conformist, desiring to meet accepted standards of behavior in their circle, and they sought to make a good impression on acquaintances. The child was regarded as one of the attributes of social well-being, to be demonstrated in society as a symbol of success.

In contrast to the public side, the family's private side reflected narrow and conservative attitudes. People were valued only on the basis of their financial status and social level, and all contacts were maintained on the basis of how others could help them succeed. Friendliness and sympathetic attitudes were insincerely expressed. These same people were perceived differently depending on any change in their social status at any given time. They said one thing to somebody's face, and another behind somebody's back. They were essentially superficial families, lacked imagination, and were highly dependent on social approval. They were pseudo-intellectuals, subject to mass-media influences. Perhaps their most important limitation was that they were incapable of expressing feelings of love to one another.

A double standard was introduced to the children from their very beginning, consisting of learning the skill to tell not what they really thought, but to express themselves only in an acceptable, conforming manner. Insincerity and hypocrisy were stressed. Parental values were centered around professional, technocratic interests without any concern for human, social and cultural values. In essence, humanistic values were absent. Typically a collection of books of prestigious writers was present, but practically never read. Children were required to study music or to participate in some dramatic or literary group — the main interest was not to further their children's education, but to seek the prestige gained through their children's achievements.

The girls felt that they were not sincerely loved and that they were unwanted by the parents as real and valued human beings. They believed that they came to be a symbol of their parent's needs. The girls also felt as if they had no spontaneity, that they were programmed to act by their parents. They lacked empathy and emotional ties with parents, resulting in a strong feeling of emotional depravation.

5. The fifth group (7% of the women) included patients who came from a family situation which, from their period of early childhood, could be described as relatively good. It was impossible to discover any obvious negative factors. The parents loved their children, took care of them, and empathized with them. The girls shared their joys and sorrows with their parents, discussed different problems, plans and troubles. Generally, parental attitudes toward alcohol were strongly negative, involving a preoccupation with seeing alcohol as "a great evil." They were intolerant of people who used alcohol. Even people who drank rarely or on special occasions were considered to be drunkards. In these families conversations about the danger of alcoholism and alcohol-related problems in society often took place. In all of these cases the parents stuck to their extreme anti-alcohol opinions, often demanding the introduction of total prohibition.

The psychological evaluation of these women revealed that they had very radical conservative attitudes toward many social problems. It was expressed, for example, in distinct divisions that all phenomena were either "bad" or "good," or "black" or "white." They attached great importance to prohibition, restrictions and penalties. The childhood experience of such children represented a combination of overprotection with elements of premature responsibility and excessive demands. The performance of school tasks, their daily timetable, and spare time were strictly controlled. It was important to get excellent marks in all subjects, to be involved in social activity, and to do well in all their undertakings. There was always a push to become better, to be the best they could be.

6. The last group consisted of 10 cases (6% of the women) coming from families where the influence of the mother was extremely

dominate in relation to their children. The husbands of these women lived independently, they did not let their wives into their spheres of interests, did not assume any responsibility for the home, or were formally divorced. These men were characterized as highly intellectual, they liked nature, hunting, participated in expeditions, climbed mountains, and floated on rafts. The interviews revealed that in all these cases the girls developed a positive idealization of their fathers. They wanted to be like them — courageous, brave, and capable of enduring any difficulties. These fantasies occurred even when the father was physically absent or only periodically present.

PSYCHOSOCIAL DEVELOPMENT

Among members of the first type or group, development was characterized by intellectual, emotional, and social immaturity. Although they achieved well academically in school, they nevertheless failed to develop a general sense of sophistication, being specifically unconcerned about cultural values. Their interests were limited and they showed no concern for intellectual matters. In a word, they were shallow. Moreover, they appeared to show little motivation to expand their horizons.

They read little, describing it as hard and boring, and tended to experience unpleasant emotional reactions when reading fiction. At home they preferred to amuse themselves by watching trivial films on TV, or chat with girlfriends. They especially liked rhythmic rock music. Their interests developed in conformance with contemporary fads. In childhood, and especially during adolescence, they showed a particularly strong tendency toward a need to form hero-images, such as film-stars, popular rock singers, or bards.

This group also typified little interest in accomplishing anything. The primary thing that they wanted was a desire for a carefree life and to be constantly happy, without putting forth any effort. Ethical and moral standards were superficial and weakly developed. Moral responsibility, the necessity to keep promises and to meet their responsibilities were lacking. They were sexually active, based more on urge than on romantic attachment. Their creed was to live for only today and not to think about the future.

Their behavior was mainly chaotic, and chiefly motivated by a need to derive pleasure. Their behavior became predictable. They repeatedly invested a large amount of energy in seeking good times, smoking and drinking, and chatting. For amusement they skipped classes, did not prepare homework, and cheated on teachers and parents. They did not experience guilt, and a fear of punishment was absent. They were governed more by gratification of an immediate need than by concern with any long term consequences of their behavior. All this behavior was, in varying degrees, a function of their family situation.

The development of the women in the second group, who came from antisocial backgrounds, was also intellectually and socially immature. Their interests in understanding such things as cultural norms, current events and personal hygiene were minimal. The interests they developed were expressions of their parents' values, and did not contain any independent thinking. In many cases the women were fearful of their parents' reaction to any assertive behavior they may have shown. Members of this group had constant nightmares. In 5 cases enuresis nocturnal occurred early in their development, and lasted till the age of 12. Intellectual and social development lagged. They received little sympathy or empathy from their parents. Their own empathic skills developed poorly; they could not imagine how others felt and expressed little compassion for relatives and friends. In brief, their behavior was largely egotistical.

This same group experienced extreme stress in their families, which was reflected in repeated fights and beatings by their mothers and fathers. This constant struggle led to situations in which they wanted to be at home as rarely as possible, especially when the father was drunk. These young girls usually made friends with girls with similar backgrounds. This behavior, on the whole, was quite close to the behavior observed in the first group, whose members were brought up with minimal parental supervision, but whose parents were not antisocial.

The members of the second group, however, showed elements of antisocial attitudes expressed in rudeness, and in extremely impulsive behavior. During their childhood they were witnesses to drinking-bouts and sexual excesses at home, and as a consequence they also manifested early sexual involvement. They seemed to have particularly sought relations with much older men as well as, with boys of the same age. One of the peculiarities of their behavior was that they often committed criminal offenses which were expressed in hooliganism, assaults in company of friends on weaker people for the purpose of beating them up, and theft of money or valuable things. They were, in some cases, involved in burglaries, sometimes in the homes of their acquaintances. Their interest in the use of mind-altering substances occurred rather early, about 12 years of age on the average, and great significance was attached to the achievement of the kef effect along with a desire to escape from reality.

The women who constituted the third group, who were brought up in orphanages or other institutional settings, developed survival skill to adapt to their severe conditions. They quickly learned to relate effectively to their peers and to younger children. They also learned very quickly that they were different from, or at a disadvantage to, children who had parents. The tutors and teachers were not accepted as substitute parents, which was largely connected with their insensitive treatment. Their main authoritative figures became older girls, who were leaders of informal groups.

The instructions and orders of the leaders were implicitly followed without any trace of protest. The habits, virtues, and intellectual opinions of the leaders were assumed as their own in a very short period of time. On the whole, the psychological dynamics of these groups were clearly defined because each of the groups' members emulated the leader, and blindly followed her lead. There was also a tendency to depend on the leader for everything, and criticism of the leader was practically absent. The group was built on the principle of a hierarchic pyramid with various levels of subordination and with strict distribution of roles. The girls tried to convey the impression that they were older, sexually appealing, and that they had sexual relations, had no fear, and were resolute and determined. All these behaviors reflected the patterns of behavior of the leaders. The group members imposed their own order in the institution, while ignoring instructions from the administration. A clear demarcation between members of these groups and outsiders was apparent. The members of the group manifested aggressiveness to nonmembers or tried to avoid contact with them. Membership in these group had high value. The members of these groups regarded themselves as being more important than those who were outside of the group. Smoking and use of alcohol were identified with maturity. Alcohol and cigarettes were used as symbols of the status of a modern woman. The customs included using slang in conversations between members, which was not used when in contact with adults. Many neologisms referring to specific styles of dress and food were also popular. Their slang contained several expressions signifying various types of alcohol beverages and drugs, with some terms representing states that developed during alcohol bouts and periods of drug-taking.

Conversations about topics of attachment, love or emotional vulnerability were not popular. The frequency of sexual intercourse and variety of partners was considered to be a symbol of superiority. Prostitution was considered as advantageous because it was the most simple and best way to earn money. Cynical, exclusively materialistic attitudes to the values of life were formed. Contacts with criminal offenders often occurred. Most of the girls bore solitude with difficulty, even during short periods. Their ability to discriminate between imagination and reality became impaired — in imagination the girls wanted to be alone (which was difficult to achieve in the institutional setting), but in reality, when this possibility was achieved, they quickly became sick and tired of it.

Any group member, with the exclusion of the leaders, who attempted to be successful in school was admonished, mocked, and even treated with hostility. What they desired instead was to live free of responsibility and to receive gratification by any means.

It was not permissible to deceive or let down other members of the group, especially those who were on the higher hierarchical level, but this loyalty did not exist beyond the group. Truthfulness and loyalty were also important within groups. The girls did not consider the use of alcohol and other drugs as a behavior which might be condemned. They considered the use of alcohol and drugs as an integral part of their life, which was in opposition to the administration's standards. They thought that through the use of alcohol and other drugs they could achieve liberation from social controls.

The women in the fourth group, who were brought up in an upward mobile environment, developed under normal living conditions and did not experience economic difficulty. As a result of their developmental experiences they showed a feeling of superiority when compared to many girls of the same age from different backgrounds. They were acquainted with and had more or less close relations only with boys and girls within their circle. The contacts always depended on the social status of their friends. It was significant to have new, fashionable clothes, books written by prestigious authors, albums of art, and video tapes with popular rock singers. The girls liked to convey their wealth and were very happy when they could show new purchases to friends which aroused envy.

It was found that these women lacked spiritual values. They were superficially informed about many matters, and lacked an interest to deepen their knowledge. Their success at school was usually good, largely motivated out of a sense of competition. They were mainly interested in looking ahead to a profitable marriage. Some of these girls were extroverted, some introverted, but both types shared a common trait — the absence of genuine interest to essential human problems, to the drama and tragedies of everyday life. They had a weak sense of compassion, and they were not concerned with suffering of others, even intimate friends.

Members of the fifth group demonstrated an early sense of responsibility that was connected with a fear of being judged by others as unworthy. They were well dressed, had a strict timetable for learning, work and spare time, and went to bed and got up as their parents required. The girls attached great importance to social activities and carried out their obligations very seriously. Their marks at school were excellent, the instructions and opinions of teachers were accepted without critical evaluation. Independent interests were not clearly defined, everything was made in accordance with instructions and programs. For example, reading of fiction was restricted only to school assignments. Their attitudes toward reality were on the whole parochial, which corresponded to the attitudes expressed at school and at home. In their world, everything was divided into opposites and existed as either black or white without any shades of meaning. All that would not correspond to this simple scheme was rejected as atypical. These girls listened only to classical music, and accepted only realistic paintings. Alcohol was identified as evil, and people who used alcohol were alcoholics. According to their opinion alcoholism was not a disease, it represented a vice caused by lack of will power. The use of alcohol was regarded as a sign of moral deficiency caused by evil influences.

Their view of the world was formed primarily by the influence of family and school. They were not exposed to broader experiences upon which to expand their frame of reference. Their time was structured so that there was no possibility to break out of the cycle of family and school relations. Their limited view of the world was to prove to be an important factor later in their lives because it could not be sustained when they were confronted with new demands, or if their views were challenged. For example, when they met new people who had opposing views, they abandoned their habitual orthodox thinking and were quick to accept the new view because they had no real basis to counter the new ideas. They thus proved to be highly susceptible to the influence of other views, no matter how extreme, even if it meant going against their original ideas. What was once considered to be strongly prohibited, such as drinking, now became extremely attractive. It was very difficult to find a new middle ground because their orthodoxy did not permit compromise to be made.

ADDICTIVE AND ANTISOCIAL BEHAVIORS

The developmental backgrounds and psychosocial characteristics described above were obtained from in-depth interviews of women with addictive and deviant behavior disorders. Based on an analysis of the attributes described, it seemed reasonable to divide all the patients into two primary groups based on the intensity of patterns of addictive and antisocial behavior.

1. Predominately Addictive Behavior

One group of women (n = 56) was identified as manifesting various types of addictive behavior. They showed a specific propensity to consume alcohol or to use other mind-altering drugs.

All the women who showed predominately addictive behavior misused alcohol. They revealed symptoms of psychological and physical dependency. Surprisingly, in almost all of the cases, involved drinking did not begin in childhood or adolescence, but only after age 25. It was found that in this group the desire to drink had a clear connection with current troubles, unpleasant situations, or emotional trauma. Most typical alcohol misuse occurred during an emotional experience caused by an unfortunate love experience, unfaithfulness or adultery. Other drinking started after the death of an intimate friend or relative, and was associated with sorrow and loneliness.

The women in this group had difficulty controlling strong negative feelings, coping with anxiety, and felt a sense of helplessness. They used alcohol as a remedy that eliminated these emotional troubles, i.e., as a form of self-medication. In some cases drinking was not related to a significant psychological event, but rather to low frustration tolerance. Many women in this group had experienced various disorders in their family life. Thirty-five were unmarried, five had never been married, and 18 were divorced. In six cases the divorce was connected with their husbands' drunkenness. In seven cases the women themselves were problem drinkers. These women indicated that they began to drink in connection with their husband's drinking—they did it "just to spite him," or in order for him to drink less. After some time they began to drink alone or with girlfriends, and lost interest in work and home duties. Interestingly, the husbands divorced their wives because they did not tolerate their wives drinking bouts while they were drinking.

Most of the married women described their husbands negatively, attaching attention to such traits as stubbornness, dullness, rudeness, ignorance, hypocrisy, insincerity, cowardice, lacking in initiative, and as being too dependent. In 12 cases the women reported that their husbands were sexually impotent and that this caused difficulty in their marriage.

Six women, ranging in age from 50 to 60, did not report abusing alcohol until late in their life. Their motivation to drink was explained by a feeling of emptiness and impossibility to devote themselves to some occupation. Their alcohol abuse coincided with retirement or with serious changes in family relations connected with separation from children, or the death of a husband. These women stressed that they were very sensitive about change in their customary style of life and disturbances in their traditions. (The possibility of misuse of alcohol in older-aged women must be taken into consideration, especially in cases involving psychiatric problems, anxiety, depression, hypochondriacal fixations and other forms of disorder.) All of these older women used alcohol at home alone, or in the company of old close friends who had common psychological problems.

2. Predominately Antisocial Behavior

The second group consisted of women with mainly antisocial behavior problems that included disorders of ethic and moral delinquency, exaggerated hedonistic lifestyles, promiscuity, and a need to obtain stimulation through self-induced acts such as drinking or drug use, or through group activity such as taking part in gang-related behaviors. The addictive behavior that these clinical patients showed was only part of a larger set of symptoms, all representative of what we consider to be deviant or antisocial behavior. Antisocial behavior is a subcategory of deviant behavior. The many different stressful situations in society all serve to contribute to the occurrence of deviant behavior.

The psychological investigation of women with predominantly addicted behavior revealed that their scores on the Male/Female MMPI Scale were lower than the norms for the standardization group. The scores were also lower than the score found for women in the group with predominantly antisocial behavior. This low score could be interpreted as reflecting a predominate image of female passivity and submissiveness. Consistently, in all the cases the women did report a strong identification with the traditional female role. All the women in this group did not clearly remember their first experience with alcohol.

An investigation by Zavjalov (1981) of addictive motivation showed that ataractical motivations (using alcohol for its relaxing, calming effect) prevailed. Although the use of alcohol did not cause euphoric or significant kef effects, most of the women said that alcohol calmed them down and made them sleepy, helped to lessen their problems, and to reduce stress. They seemed to be aware before they started drinking that alcohol would have such effects.

Among the cases showing ataractical motivation other addictive motivation was also registered in the form of seeking to isolate themselves. For example, one of the patients revealed the following: "I drink in order to protect myself from tiresome fusses, talk, gossip, and all this flow of information. Often I came home already drunk to go to bed and do not utter a word to anybody." As a rule alcohol was used alone and it was often concealed from relatives and friends. Women drank comparatively high doses of alcohol in relatively short-time intervals. There were few tendencies to experience prolonged drinking-bouts. The women tried to achieve desirable effects as fast as possible, to lose themselves, and to forget their troubles and unpleasant thoughts — they sought to think nothing.

This style of drinking led to relatively fast development of alcohol dependence, first psychological, then physical. We noted that in most cases the first signs of physical dependency were symptoms of withdrawal, but the symptoms of loss of control did not develop or occurred very much later. Their MMPI profiles were consistent with symptoms of neurosis, hypochondria and depression.

In some cases the patients used not only alcohol, but also barbiturates and tranquilizers for similar purposes — to achieve psychological relaxation. Drugs were taken in the evenings or nights, and in many cases this was connected with difficulty getting alcohol beverages. Many of these patients reported that it was too much for them to go to the store and stand in a queue to get alcohol. Subsequently, in some cases, psychological and physical dependency to drugs developed. After they started using other drugs their interest in alcohol lessened because it was considered to be a weak remedy in comparison to the effects of other drugs. Their motivation for using drugs also changed from ataractic motives to hedonistic ones. The women not only wanted to be relaxed, but also sought to indulge in daydreams and revelry, and to seek an escape from reality by withdrawing into fantasies.

Many of the women used alcohol without clearly connecting it with psychotraumatic events. The urge to use alcohol was directly related to other motivation — alcohol was used for the purpose of achieving euphoria, increasing fantasies, changing one's perception of reality, to see everything better than it was, to be able to remember something very pleasant which was forgotten long ago, and to withdraw into oneself. In all these cases a deep appreciation of alcohol's effect took place. These women connected alcohol with its unusual capacity to change one's state of consciousness. Experiences of this type were probably associated with an ability for self-suggestion. MMPI data noted for these patients consisted of high scores on the HY and MF scales. The women were characterized by adventurousness, impulsiveness, and extravagant behavior.

Further study of these women discovered that their hedonistic motivation to drink or use other drugs was primarily connected with an attempt to alter their consciousness. While in a state of light alcohol intoxication and in company of friends, these women felt themselves to be exciting, lively, attractive, and interested in other people. In conversations they were witty and sarcastic. Sometimes they wanted to escape from society and kefed alone. The women in this group had some interest in the drugs with psychotropic effects, such as hashish or tranquilizers, but they had no interest in hard drugs such as organic solvents.

One of the peculiarities of this group of women was their comparatively high psychic and motor activity. In childhood they attracted attention to themselves by restless behavior, capriciousness, and constant but not productive activity. They did not like to play with dolls or play house with other girls. They preferred to play with boys, take part in hooliganism, run on the streets, set fire to the post boxes, ruin lifts, and make obscene graffiti. They did not complete their homework, missed classes, and frequently deceived their parents and teachers. At the same time they tried to make a good impression on adults, attempting to demonstrate their independence and cleverness to evoke interest in themselves. In adolescents the girls were coquettish, flirtatious, and tried to dress fashionably. They lacked interest in their home life. Staying at home caused boredom and psychological discomfort. They liked to be in company with others who shared similar interests who were themselves unstable. Every group had favorite places to meet to spend their free time together.

During the summer the girls preferred to stay on the streets in the central part of Novosibirsk, near hotels, restaurants, parks, or around the railroad station or docks. As a rule every group had its own place, usually near their homes. In winter the girls gathered in their friends flats when parents were absent, or sometimes gathered in cellars and attics.

Hedonistic motivations prevailed. They were preoccupied with a need to satisfy their desires immediately without thinking about any unpleasant consequences. Thought about punishment were minimal and they did not hold back impulsive behavior. The need for stimulation prevailed. The girls had numerous sexual contacts with teenagers and unknown men. In some cases girls visited places in which antisocial personalities gathered. The contrast between their home and family conditions and the situations in which the girls functioned was very dramatic.

The promiscuity, in many cases, could not be explained as just satisfying a need for sexual gratification. Psychological studies indicated that their early sexual behavior represented deeper disorders, which was not only tied to a desire for gratification, but with a strong urge to experience unusual and risky situations. It was found that most of their sexual contacts were not gratifying unless it occurred in an unusual or risky context.

All these women had sexual experiences before 18 years, and the younger ones did not want to marry. Some of the reasons for not wanting to marry were: "The family is burdensome," "As yet I am not satisfied with boys," "I feel only a desire for new experiences." They saw men as a sexual objects first, and as companions or lovers as second. Most of the older single women did not feel any regret about not having married. The married patients displayed irresponsibility about family matters, were not able to experience comfort at home, or organize the household. They were also irresponsible with respect to caring for their children.

The women with antisocial behavior were in constant conflict with many people, especially members of their family. They did not understand the rights of other people, could not empathize with others, and they tended to exploit all of their relatives. The ability to sustain sincere emotional relationships was absent, people were used as objects. Only their own desires and emotions were accepted. Anxiety was usually absent, they did not feel guilt or show remorse.

MMPI data showed higher MF scale scores in contrast to the low scores obtained by women with predominantly addictive behavior. The antisocial women were indifferent to traditional female values.

Low frustration tolerance was expressed, delay of satisfaction of their wishes was impossible. All aims were momentary or short-coming. Their behavior was characterized by an immediate need to satisfy impulses and to achieving pleasure at any cost. There were elements of hysteria in difficult situations, a tendency to lie, to accuse others and to stress their own innocence.

Some of these women conveyed a good impression during the clinical interviews. They told stories about their good relations with people, with family members; they were informal and witty. Other women were dysphoric, angry, impudent. Some of them were often in conflict with the law because of thefts or hooliganism.

Others expressed less antisocial behavior in comparison to others. These women held jobs for long periods of time, usually in fields where close and long contacts with the same people were not necessary. However, even in these cases interpersonal relations in families were distorted. Serious relations with people did not form. People around them got tired, frustrated and eventually were fed up with being treated as objects.

A basic motive common to all these women with predominantly antisocial behavior was a desire to receive pleasure. Some of them strived to place themselves in risky situations, to experience unusual events — they enjoyed feeling a sense of danger. The use of alcohol and drugs was accepted as a means of inducing a pleasurable state. Most of the women in the group with predominant antisocial behavior used alcohol without dependency. They had rather high alcohol tolerance and drank without severe alcohol intoxication. None of these women could remember any details about their first drinking experiences, or whether it elicited a strong positive or negative effect. Later, when their addictive behavior was formed it was not only attributable to the pharmacological effects of alcohol, but also to a complex situation involving association with other drinkers and sexual partners. Their drinking or drug use, however, did not attain a level where it impaired their level of functioning.

No data about the ataractic or kef effects of alcohol were obtained. The women said that alcohol did not cause significant changes of their mental state, did not help to significantly increase or decrease their activity levels, did not stimulate imagination, or interfere with their ability to dream. Their primary motive for drinking was to experience alcohol's disinhibition effect, especially among the women who gambled.

Hedonistic motivation prevailed in many cases among women in the predominately addictive group. Some of these women remembered their first drinking experiences long after they had occurred. For them, alcohol, when they started to drink, induced development of a very pleasant state, which was expressed in the following terms: "uplifting," "magnificent," "in paradise," "happiness," or "gay." Some of them said, "I'd like to dance, sing, make something unusual." These positive reactions, however, diminished rather quickly.

Despite the psychopharmacological effect of alcohol, even these women did not strive to drink alone, without company. Alcohol was used in company of friends. The alcohol itself, however, was as important as the pleasure experienced by being part of a group. Usually relatively small amounts of alcohol were consumed, which did not cause intoxication, but which induced a mild euphoric effect.

A small number of these women not only used alcohol, but also other mind-altering drugs, including hashish, tranquilizers, cyclodol and demerol. In these cases their motives for drug use was similar to the drug-effect motive described by Segal et al. (1982). The drug-effect motive described by Segal et al., represented a need to use drugs to expand one's self awareness and to achieve new and different experiences. Our patients seemed to be primarily more interested in satisfying a need for new and different experiences rather than in expanding their self-awareness.

Among a few women the use of alcohol was connected with a desire to obtain a kef effect, associated with increased imagination (dreamy states, reveries). In these cases the women showed a strong desire to be left alone, they became irritable when around other people. The kef effect of alcohol in these women occurred when they were in the company of persons of the same sex. In other cases, typical euphoric or ataractic effects occurred. (We separated these and other effects of alcohol in a previous investigation [Korolenko & Botchkareva, 1982].) When they drank their desire to be coquettish increased. They indicated that their mood while drinking was dependent on their state of mind before drinking. ("If I'm well, so after drink I will be better." "If I'm bad alcohol did not change how I felt.") Although alcohol could increase their basic mood, it only had a small effect on changing its contents. For example, if alcohol was used because the drinker felt irritable, unhappy, insulted, all of these states were aggravated after drinking and caused conflict with other people. What was most interesting, however, was that these women were usually in a good mood whether they were drinking or not.

Some women with antisocial behavior used alcohol because of the influence of others. Their early drinking occurred in company of men and women who abused alcohol intensively, and they soon learned to imitate their behavior. They took part in drinking in such groups two to three times a week. Most of these groups included men who abused alcohol.

On the average, after five years of such drinking, physical dependence developed. The appearance of physical dependence was expressed by a loss of control, which totally changed their behavior, and the onset of the withdrawal syndrome. The basic elements of antisocial behavior, however, continued to be expressed. In many cases the women changed friends because of conflicts about their excessive drinking during drinking episodes. These conflicts were connected with their unacceptable behavior while drinking together, largely as a result of their loss of control. After they drank to the point of severe intoxication they were unable to function and could not return home without the help of other people. These women, in contrast to women who drank alcoholically without manifesting severe antisocial behavior, had no symptoms of inferiority feelings, and typical intervals between alcohol excesses were absent. The socially deviant women were indifferent to being humiliated by their friends when deeply intoxicated.

Some women, who drank little and did not use other drugs, showed a marked interest in gambling. The gambling developed as a part of their antisocial behavior. Antisocial behaviors were also expressed in promiscuity, aggressiveness, and vagrancy. Their gambling was strongly reinforced in the groups to which they belonged. Their gambling was also motivated by a need to pay creditors, which also led to criminal acts and, in some cases, to prostitution. The gambling was usually connected with the use of alcohol during the games, which was an acceptable standard. A tendency to use alcohol beyond the gambling situation was not expressed.

Although we studied the drinking behavior of women in the two different groups, one which consisted of women who were predominately addicted, and the other consisting of women who were predominately antisocial, the women in both groups also expressed reasons for not drinking—reasons we termed as negative motives. But despite these negative motives the women continued to drink. These negative motives, however, were mostly associated with women with predominately addictive behavior. The reasons for not drinking that were most often expressed among these were: "I'm afraid to become alcoholic," "a fear of losing social acceptance," "to be accused by relatives, parents, or authoritative people." In some cases negative motivations were connected with financial reasons—it cost too much for them to drink.

The negative motivations in women with predominantly antisocial behavior appeared less frequently. Expressed most often was "to avoid trouble with police," followed by "not wanting to pay money for alcohol."

Some of the women who manifested gambling disorders indicated that although they did drink they were nevertheless afraid that they would lose control and be unable to gamble well.

CONCLUSIONS

As a result of our studies the concept of addictive behavior as a part of deviant behavior was introduced, and some types of these behaviors were analyzed in women. Two groups of women were identified: (1) women with predominant addictive behavior, and (2) women with predominant antisocial behavior. Addictive behavior was expressed in various forms: misuse of alcohol, use of mind-altering drugs and toxic substances or gambling. Antisocial behavior was characterized by violations of social and moral values, lack of emotional attachment to parents, relatives and friends, promiscuity, and criminality.

The significance of different types of upbringing in the occurrences of addictive and antisocial behavior was established. Antisocial behavior was connected, as a rule, with neglectful families who rejected their children; alcoholism and criminal behavior by parents were common. The children's antisocial behavior occurred early in childhood and imitated their parental attitudes. Development in upward mobile families without spiritual values, in families with extreme attitudes, and teetotaler attitudes, lead to the development of predominantly antisocial and predominantly addictive behavior.

An analysis of motivations for using alcohol or drugs showed that in the predominantly addictive group ataractical motivation and a need to alter consciousness (expanded awareness) prevailed. In the predominantly antisocial group, hedonistic and ataractic motives prevailed.

Gambling, as an addictive behavior, was more prominent in women with antisocial behavior and was combined with a tendency to criminality when compared to women manifesting addictive behavior.

Information was also obtained about the significance of stress in the development of addictive behavior of women. It was found that such factors as divorces, loneliness, and dissatisfaction in one's professional career may be significant.

The development of an effective prevention program will, to a large degree, depend on a complex interaction involving an understanding of predominately addictive behavior and predominately antisocial behavior as different forms of deviant behavior. Special significance also needs to be given to understanding the backgrounds of people who develop deviant behaviors.

Treatment needs to be based on helping patients in developing effective relationships with other people instead of maintaining pathological interactions in which they relate to people as objects.

LIST OF REFERENCES

Korolenko, C. P. & Bochkareva, N. L. (1982). *Peculiarities of certain exogenetic intoxications under the northern conditions.* Novosibirsk, USSR: Science Press.

Korolenko, C. P., & Timofeeva, A. S. (1986). *The roots of alcoholism.* Novosibirsk, USSR: Books Edition.

Segal, B., Cromer, F., Hobfoll, S., & Wasserman, P. Z. (1982). Patterns of reasons for drug use among detained and adjudicated juveniles. *The International Journal of the Addictions, 17*(7), 1117-1130.

Segal, B. (1988). *Drugs and behavior*. New York: Gardner Press.

Zavjalov, V. (1981) *Clinical and psychological study of some formation mechanism of alcohol dependence*. Unpublished Dissertation, Novosibirsk.

The "Rapid Course of Development" of Early Alcoholism in Young People

A. Dragun, MD

INTRODUCTION

The climatic and geographical peculiarities, intensity of industrial and economic development in Siberia, accompanied by the process of urbanization and sharp changes in the demographical situation during the last three decades, requires that attention be given to how people adjust to a stressful environment. These conditions, which exert a severe strain on people's adaptation capabilities, may contribute to shortening the length of time it takes for development of alcohol dependence, as well as impact its features and prevalence rates (Korolenko & Bochkarjova, 1982).

Historically established in Siberia was a style of intensive drinking which was characterized primarily by consuming large amounts of alcohol (chiefly vodka) or home-brewed whiskey. It should be noted, however, that in spite of this drinking style the alcohol problem rate remained fairly low. This low rate of problem-drinking can be explained mainly by the presence of a rigid system of traditions and rituals connected with drinking in the community and within the family. The frequency of drinking and the reasons for it was firmly restricted to religious feasts and to family occasions; drinking while working was strongly condemned. As a rule, in each village there were two or three hard drinkers whose individual drinking patterns caused numerous alcohol-related problems. Their behavior served as negative role-models for the children in the com-

A. Dragun is affiliated with the Department of Psychiatry, Novosibirsk Medical Institute.

munity. Over time, the traditional drinking style was altered by the process of migration.

The intensive migration of rural populations into cities, especially during the past 30 years, resulted in significant disruptions in family relationships, particularly among those that were traditionally patriarchal. Families also experienced a loss of some of their most significant traditions and customs, including the rituals connected with drinking. Traditional ceremonial drinking rapidly changed to frequent and uncontrolled drinking, largely as a function of stress arising from having to meet the new demands made by living in an urban environment. As a function of urbanization people were subjected to bureaucracy and new cultural traditions. Much of their energy was invested into adapting to their new situation. Frustration and stress became an every day experience, and these contributed to an increase in drinking. This drinking rapidly developed into alcohol abuse and development of alcohol addiction. Prevalence levels for alcohol-related problems increased accordingly.

One popular theory advanced by the medical community to account for this increase in problem drinking was that it was due to some form of psycho-organic disorders induced by abusing alcohol. This approach failed to account for any social-psychological factors that may have been involved. Research by Korolenko (1978) indicated that the psycho-organic model was an insufficient explanation to account for the drinking behavior exhibited by these new arrivals. Korolenko argued that dependence on alcohol was a direct function of the amount and frequency of drinking, and that there was a legitimate need to understand that dependence on alcohol involved both psychological and physical dependence. This approach not only accounts for the medical aspects of alcoholism, but also allows for an understanding of the significance of social, psychological and biological factors in the development of alcoholism.

The purpose of the present research was to study the dynamics and features of the *Rapid Onset of Early Alcoholism* and the significance of certain socio-psychological factors in its formation in young adults.

METHOD

The study began with 340 industrial workers, all men, aged 18 to 30 years, who were clinically diagnosed as alcoholic. All were interviewed with respect to their drinking behavior, and, an in-depth interview of each of the men focused on obtaining information about their psychological problems. Other information was also obtained about their physical status. A history of their drinking and family relationship was also derived. Special emphasis was placed on obtaining information about their childhood development, parental relationships, family drinking rituals, and any behavioral deviations, including criminal behavior.

In accordance with the purposes of the present research, any patients that showed signs of neuroses, psychopathic tendencies, serious physical or mental pathology, or brain damage were excluded from the study. Those patients who were diagnosed as being only psychologically dependent on alcohol were also excluded. The purpose of screening these cases was to identify a clinical group of men who were physically dependent on alcohol, and who did not use other drugs.

As a result of the screening process, 117 patients formed the basic study group. Information was obtained about their motives for drinking and their personality characteristics using the Cattell 16 PF Scale. These men were also observed in relationship to their drinking behavior over a period of 2.5 to three years.

The data was analyzed to determine if any differences could be identified with respect to the length of development of the onset of alcohol withdrawal syndrome. Two groups were identified. One group (Group A) consisted of 67 patients who showed a rapid course of early alcoholism, and who evidenced withdrawal after three years from the onset of regular drinking. A second group (Group B) consisted of 50 patients who did not evidence withdrawal symptoms during this three year period.

The mean age of the workers in Group A was 20.9 years, ranged from 19 to 26. For Group B, the mean age was 23.7 years and ranged from 21 to 27. Both groups were comparable with respect to education levels, professional and marital status.

All the cases started to drink regularly after 18 years of age. The mean age for Group A was 20 years, and 20.1 years for Group B.

At the beginning of the present investigation all patients manifested signs of physical alcohol dependence: a craving for alcohol to achieve its desired effects and a fixation on alcohol.

RESULTS

1. Background Factors

The study of background factors found that in Group A (the rapid onset group) there was a significant relationship between a rapid course and a family history of alcoholism ($p = < 0.01$). A significant relationship was also found between the rapid course and fathers' drinking ($p = < 0.02$) and between intense parental conflict ($p = < 0.01$). Further relationships were also found between rapid course and mood alteration during the first contact with alcohol and retained reminiscences about it ($p = < 0.02$). An association was also found between rapid course and frequent conflicts with parents and teachers while in school ($p = < 0.05$).

The results of investigation of family history of alcoholism and mental illness are presented in Table 1.

Intensive conflict in parental relationships was revealed in 22 patients in Group A (32.8%) and by 6 patients in Group B (12.0%).

TABLE 1. Family History of Alcoholism and Mental Illness in Group A and Group B

		Group A (Rapid Onset)		Group B (Longer Onset)	
		N	Percent	N	Percent
Alcoholism		41	61.1	18	36.0
Mental Illness		2	3.0	-	-
Alcoholism of:	Father	2	38.8	11	22.0
	Mother	2	3.0	-	-
	Both parents	9	13.4	4	8.0

The patients with a rapid course of early alcoholism remembered their first intoxication significantly better than members of Group B. The age and reasons for their initial drinking did not differ significantly between the groups (see Table 2). Most of the patients in either group had their first drink in their teens with peers outside of their home.

Ninety percent of the patients in Group A and 58 percent of those in Group B experienced alcohol euphoria the first time they were intoxicated and retained positive memories about it. In addition, this positive impression was reinforced by an absence of any negative physical effects during or after intoxication. It is important to note that most of the alcoholics in Group A reported that they became aware of the mind-altering effect of alcohol during their first intoxication.

An initial absence of the vomiting reflex to overdoses of alcohol was found in 34.3 percent of the patients in Group A and in 14 percent of those in Group B.

Behavioral deviations during school age years (frequent conflicts with parents and teachers, running away from home, delinquency, etc.) were found in 51 percent of the patients in Group A and in 38 percent of those in Group B. This difference was statistically significant. Significant differences, however, were not found between the two groups with respect to the frequency of parental drinking or antisocial (i.e., criminal acts) behavior.

2. Motives for Drinking

The motives for drinking varied considerably in each group. Members of Group B conveyed motives that represented an exaggerated intention to follow social rituals connected with drinking, the seeking of broader social occasions for drinking, and to maintain social relationships. Members of Group A had difficulty expressing their motives for drinking or gave rather elusive, traditional reasons, such as drinking on weekends, drinking to celebrate holidays, or because it is just the thing to do.

A more detailed inquiry of those in Group A found that they drank alcoholically but were unaware of why they drank so heavily. Drinking was considered to be an accepted activity in a special so-

TABLE 2. Age, Reasons for and Situation of First Contact with Alcohol in Basic and Control Groups

	Basic Group		Control Group	
	N	Percent	N	Percent
Age before 10	2	3.0	3	6.0
10 - 13	5	7.5	6	12.0
14 - 16	47	70.1	31	62.0
17 - 20	13	19.4	10	20.0
Reasons:				
Social holidays and family occasions	30	44.7	22	44.0
Influence of company	16	23.9	12	24.0
Intention to be "an adult man"	6	9.0	8	16.0
"Alcohol" traditions	5	7.5	-	-
Curiosity	3	4.5	6	12.0
Influence of adults	3	4.5	2	4.0
"First pay"	3	4.5	-	-
Didn't remember	1	1.5	-	-
Situation:				
Ritual, at home	3	4.5	3	6.0
Ritual, outside of the home	5	7.5	5	10.0
Accidental, outside of the home	59	88.0	42	84.0
Settings:				
of peers	54	80.5	43	86.0
of adults	6	9.0	2	4.0
mixed	5	7.5	5	10.0
in isolation	2	3.0	-	-

cial environment, which was usually restricted to other drinking partners. Their association with other drinkers during most of their free time prevented them from engaging in other activities with nondrinking partners.

Twenty-four percent of the patients in Group A and 26 percent in Group B displayed ataractic (anxiety-reducing) motives for drinking, usually characterized by a desire to reduce psycho-emotional stress, digress from troubles, resolve emotional problems and personal conflicts, and to help cope with fear, anxiety, depression and feelings of guilt. Such use can be referred to as drinking to self-medicate oneself, which was more typical for group B. The patients in Group A reported that they drank primarily to cope with free-floating anxiety.

A hedonistic motive, characterized by a craving to achieve pleasure from alcohol intoxication, was expressed by 18 percent of the members of Group A, and by 16 percent in Group B. It should be noted that in Group B the patients associated the desire for obtaining pleasure not only with the alcohol itself but also with the companionship involved in drinking. They were particularly sensitive to the context in which drinking took place and the nature of their relationship with their friends. In contrast, those in Group A oriented themselves more to the general effects of alcohol.

Motives equivalent to sensation seeking (Segal, 1988) were registered in both groups. These motives reflected a striving to obtain a high level of stimulation with the intent to escape from boredom and inaction.

A small number of cases in both groups indicated that their drinking was largely induced or influenced by others. They described group pressure and their inability to refuse drinks as being responsible for their alcohol abuse.

3. The Dynamics of Alcohol Dependence and the Clinical Picture of Alcoholism

The dynamics and clinical picture of alcoholism in Group A had a number of special features. The rapid course of early alcoholism was manifested by a rapid development of the signs of psychological dependence. Ninety percent of the patients in Group A experienced their first intoxication (i.e., got acquainted with the psychopharmacological effects of alcohol) during their initial contact with alcohol beverages. It thus appears that their drinking behavior was shaped to a large extent by the combined effect of a rather high initial tolerance to alcohol and the desire to experience the mind-altering effects of alcohol.

In contrast to Group A, members of group B manifested episodic drinking, which was largely influenced by their social environment, their own expectations about the effects of alcohol, and by various social rituals.

The mean length of time for symptoms of alcoholism to develop is presented in Table 3. It was found that the length time to the establishment of loss of control was significantly correlated ($p = < .05$) with the length of time for the development of all the symptoms of alcoholism. This finding suggests that early formation of loss of control (1.5 to 2 years from the onset of regular drinking) may be a sufficiently reliable predictive criterion for identifying drinkers with rapid development of alcohol dependence. It should be noted, that the amount of alcohol consumed, rather than frequency of drinking, was also found to be a strong predictor of rapid course of alcoholism.

One of the peculiarities of rapid course of alcoholism was the early formation of a tendency to primarily drink large amounts of alcohol leading to deeply intoxicated states. This tendency was established during the first months of regular drinking. Such behavior was most typical for persons who demonstrated low frustration tolerance, disturbances in social adaptation, and who expressed an intention to "forget their troubles," "escape from reality," or "lose consciousness" through drinking.

The early use of alcohol substitutes, such as medicines or industrial products containing alcohol, was typical for patients in Group A. Some even preferred alcohol substitutes to alcohol. The rapid development of deep intoxication with a specific "stupefying" effect made alcohol substitutes attractive for these patients.

In Group A, 40 percent of the patients who experienced a loss of control said that their craving for alcohol was connected with a need to reduce an unpleasant emotional condition such as anxiety or tension during intoxication. Thus their loss of control was com-

TABLE 3. Mean Length of Forming of Symptoms of Alcoholism in Basic and Control Groups from the Onset of Systematic Drinking (In Years)

	Basic Group	Control Group
Loss of control	1.4 + 0.1 (n = 67)	4.3 + 0.2 (n = 34)
Withdrawal syndrome	2.8 + 0.1 (n = 67)	5.8 + 0.2 (n = 39)
Drinking bouts	3.5 + 0.1 (n = 20)	7.2 + 0.2 (n = 12)
Alcohol amnesia	2.9 + 0.2 (n = 20)	6.9 + 0.3 (n = 12)
Use of alcohol substitutes	2.0 + 0.3 (n = 29)	6.2 + 0.5 (n = 3)

pounded by psychological factors. The remaining patients (60%) also experienced a loss of control, but did not express a craving for alcohol to reduce anxiety or tension. They drank, instead, because they could not satisfy their need for alcohol. This finding suggests that loss of control may not only be driven by physical factors, but that psychological processes are also involved and have to be taken into consideration when treating the client. Merely stopping the drinking may not be sufficient if the underlying problems are not dealt with.

4. Personality

The results of the analysis of the 16 PF are presented in Table 4. An attempt to find an overall difference in the 16 PF profiles for the two groups was unsuccessful, but scores on some of the scales differed significantly. The limited number of differences did not justify an interpretation of the findings.

DISCUSSION

This research was undertaken to identify the dynamics and features of the rapid onset of early alcoholism and the significance of certain socio-psychological factors in its formation in young male adults. An intense evaluation of men with drinking problems showed that one group followed what might be called the traditional path to alcoholism, while the other showed a more rapid development. These two groups differed with respect to their drinking behaviors and causes.

It has been shown that a family history of alcoholism is an important factor connected to the development of a rapid course of early alcoholism. The influence of social factors was also discussed, and was shown to be less significantly related.

The psycho-physiological reaction to alcohol in Group A included high susceptibility to certain psychopharmacological effects of alcohol, initial absence of vomiting reflex to overdoses of alcohol beverages, and a high initial tolerance to alcohol. It should be noted that the majority of patients in Group A experienced psychopharmacological effects of alcohol beginning with their first drinking episode. This finding supports the work of Fromme and

TABLE 4. Mean Scores and Standard Errors of 16 PF Scales in Basic and Control Groups

Scale	Basic Group (n = 56)	Control Group (n = 47)	
A	5.4 + 0.2	5.0 + 0.2	NS
B	5.9 + 0.3	5.3 + 0.3	NS
C	3.6 + 0.2	5.3 + 0.2	$p < .01$
E	4.7 + 0.3	4.6 + 0.2	NS
F	5.7 + 0.2	6.0 + 0.3	NS
G	4.4 + 0.2	5.2 ÷ 0.3	NS
H	4.8 + 0.2	5.1 + 0.3	NS
I	6.0 + 0.3	5.4 + 0.2	NS
L	7.2 + 0.2	6.0 + 0.2	$p < .01$
M	5.4 + 0.3	5.5 + 0.3	NS
N	4.5 + 0.3	5.0 + 0.4	NS
O	7.4 + 0.2	6.0 + 0.2	$p < .01$
Q1	5.9 + 0.3	5.8 + 0.3	NS
Q2	5.5 + 0.2	5.0 + 0.2	NS
Q3	5.8 + 0.3	6.9 + 0.2	$p < .05$
Q4	7.7 + 0.2	5.1 + 0.2	$p < .01$

Samson (1983), who indicated that the drinker's reaction to the pharmacological effect of alcohol itself may influence subsequent drinking. Kuehle et al. (1974) pointed out that the positive memories about one's first intoxication may be a strong predictor of development of alcoholism.

The initial high tolerance to alcohol that was observed among the men in this study is consistent with Jellinek's (1960) findings and, as he indicated, may be a predisposing factor in the development of alcohol addiction because it allows one to consume moderately large amounts of alcohol without any appreciable negative physical effects. Cahalan and Room (1974) wrote that people who experienced more negative than positive alcohol effects while intoxicated are less disposed to hard drinking.

The present findings indicate, as Battegay and Bergdol (1979) and Radonco-Thomas et al. (1980) have suggested, that the influence of family history of alcoholism includes both genetic and psychosocial factors. Alexander (1956) pointed out the importance of physiological constitution in the development of most cases of alcoholism. Goodwin et al. (1974) hold that the weighty evidence of genetic component of inheritance has been found for hard forms of alcoholism exclusively.

When considering the role of genetic factors in alcoholism, however, it is important to recognize that one's style of intensive drinking, which can be related to cultural norms, may lead to a fixation in studying past generations and on determining the inheritance of certain peculiarities of alcohol metabolism, rather than focusing on understanding the *type of alcoholism* manifested and deriving a means of treating it. Genetic factor peculiarities may or may not contribute to the development of alcohol dependence, contingent on the influence that social and psychological factors have on individual drinking patterns.

The data from the present study further demonstrate the significance of motives for drinking. As a whole the motives for drinking in the rapid development group were less conscious and differed in comparison to traditional drinkers. The motives for drinking in Group A were determined by the individual characteristics of the patients (their personality features, peculiarities of psychophysiological reaction to alcohol, etc.), rather than by a complex interaction of social factors apparent in Group B.

A shortening of the length of development of all symptoms of alcoholism was found in Group A. The early formation of loss of control was the strongest predictor of rapid development of the signs of alcohol dependence. The dynamic and clinical picture of alcoholism in Group A had a number of distinct features, including a tendency to use large amounts of alcohol and alcohol substitutes leading to deep intoxication.

The amount of alcohol consumed rather than the frequency of drinking was found to be a good predictor of rapid development of alcoholism. These results conform to the findings by Bowman et al. (1975), Wodak et al. (1983), and Vogel-Sprott et al. (1983). It is interesting to note that Parsons (1975) concluded that the cytotoxic effect of high doses of alcohol exclusively without the previous signs of psychic alcohol dependence can contribute to alcoholism. The findings from this study tends to support Parsons' conclusion.

LIST OF REFERENCES

Alexander, C. (1956). Views on the etiology of alcoholism. II. The Psychodynamic view. In Kruse (Ed.). *Alcoholism as a medical problem* (pp. 40-46).

Battegay, R., & Bergdol, A. (1979). Psychiatrische aspekte des alkoholismus: Ursachen und entstehungsbedingungen. In R. Battegay, & M. Weisser (Eds.), *Prophylaxe des alkoholismus* (pp. 94-111). Berlin: Verlag Haus Huber.

Bowman, R., Stein, L., & Newton, J. (1975). Measurement interpretation of drinking behavior. *Journal of Studies on Alcohol, 36,* 1145-1152.

Cahalan, D. & Room, R. (1974). *Problem drinking among American men.* New Brunswick, NJ: Rutgers Center of Alcohol Studies.

Korolenko, C. (1978). *Human psychophysiology in extreme conditions.* Leningrad, USSR: Medicine.

Korolenko, C., & Bochkarjova, N. (1982). *The peculiarities of some exogenous intoxications in the conditions of the far north.* Novosibirsk, USSR: Science.

Fromme, K, & Sampson, H. (1983). A survey analysis of first intoxication experiences. *Journal of Alcohol Studies, 44,* 905-910.

Goodwin, D., Schulsinger, F., & Hermansen, L. (1974). Drinking problems in adopted and nonadopted sons of alcoholics. *Archives of General Psychiatry, 31,* 164-169.

Jellinek, E. (1960). *The disease concept of alcoholism.* New Haven: Hillhouse Press.

Kuehle, J., Anderson, W., & Chandler, E. (1974). First drinking experience in addictive and nonaddictive drinkers. *Archives of General Psychiatry, 31,* 521-523.

Parsons, O. (1975). Brain damage in alcoholics: Altered states of unconsciousness. In M. Gross (Ed.), *Alcohol intoxication and withdrawal: Experimental studies* (pp. 569-584). NY: Plenum.

Redneck, S., Garcin, F., & Dewer, D. (1980). A possible "ecopharmacogenetical" model in neuropsychopharmacology aspects in alcoholism and pharmaco-dependence. *Prog. Neuro-Psychopharm*, *4*, 313-315.

Segal, B. (1988). *Drugs and behavior*. NY: Gardner Press.

Vogel-Sprott, M. (1981). Response measures of social drinking. *Journal of Studies on Alcohol*, *44*, 817-836.

Wodak, A., Saunders, J., Mensah, I., & Williams, R. (1983). Severity of alcohol dependence in patients with alcoholic liver disease. *British Medical Journal*, *287*, 1420-1422.

REVIEWS

Soviet and American Perspectives on Addiction: A Brief Critique

D. J. Lettieri, PhD

In America, at the turn of the century, alcoholism was often characterized as moral turpitude, weak character and deviant behavior. In the 1930s, alcoholism came to be viewed as a disease, in which a medical model was invoked such that the user was to be seen as a victim rather than perpetrator of the disease. In clinical practice this meant that alcoholics should receive treatment rather than retribution. The responsibility for both the problem and the solution was now placed in the hands of the care-giver rather than the alcoholic per se. Clearly, this medical view led to more humane and potentially beneficial clinical care of the alcoholic. During the 1950s, Isidor Chein's classic work, The Road to H, hallmarked the increasing rise of illicit drug use in America. At that time and up until the early 1980s, illicit drug use was often characterized as deviant behavior. This attitude persisted, in large measure, as a byproduct of the legal sanctions attached to such drug use. In the mid 1960s, Vincent Dole suggested that heroin addiction might be a metabolic deficiency, and proposed methadone as a suitable treatment regimen. The view that drug addiction might be a disease did not garner much favor with the American populace because of the crime which often attended its use. As early as 1971, one President proclaimed "war on drugs." The linkage of drug users and criminal behavior was clearly a deterrent to implementation of more medically oriented treatment regimens. To this day, many Americans still consider illicit drug use as deviant behavior. Thus in America, many of us are of two minds, illicit drug use is deviant and criminal, while abuse of legal drugs and alcohol are often seen as disease processes.

The Soviet position, as presented in these papers, characterizes alcohol and drug use as a subcategory of deviant behavior. In this regard the Soviet position is consonant with American views of illicit drug use. These theoretical positions take on significance when they help shape the conduct of clinical practice. It has often been the clinician's frustration with a particular treatment regimen that has ushered in new theoretical conceptions of addiction. For example, American clinicians, confronted with continually low addiction treatment success rates, are now proposing that one must carefully match the client with the treatment. It is no longer tenable to argue that addiction is a unidimensional phenomenon nor that one standard or generic treatment regimen can work with the vast array of addicted clients. Attendant to this is the view that there may not be a single addictive personality syndrome. In short, people take drugs to change what they see as negative emotional states. The user is often seen as his own psychopharmacologist. He uses substances to modulate his affects. These affective states may be genetically heritable, or they may be situational. It is of particular interest that some Soviet research attributes alcoholism to the extreme and harsh climatic conditions present in parts of that country. Underlying that etiological consideration is a recognition that there are many types of addictive personalities, that addiction is multidimensional, and that an array of different treatments may be needed to effectively ameliorate the addictive condition. In some circles in America, one hears talk of alcoholisms, rather than alcoholism. The Soviets, building on the work of Jellinick, have continued to recognize the multifaceted aspects of alcoholism, and clearly acknowledge a range of types of differential treatments for each of the types of alcoholic and drug addicted persons.

While Americans may be less comfortable with the view that alcoholism is a subcategory of deviance, there is some groundbreaking work that suggests the heritability of alcoholism. For example, the work of Robert Cloninger at Washington University in St. Louis, Missouri, contends that alcoholic parents may genetically transmit a trait of antisocial behavior to their offspring. As the offspring attempt to control and modify their negative, impulsive and antisocial tendencies, they soon discover that alcohol is a relatively effective medicine. Thus while no one contends there is an alcohol gene, per se, there is strong suggestive evidence for the heritability of antisocialness, which in turn can lead to excessive substance use. In this regard the American and Soviet positions may be more consonant than dissonant.

Ultimately, I suspect that the resolution of which theoretical perspective is correct will rely on the advances of clinical practice. If the careful matching of clients to treatments markedly enhances treatment success, then issues of etiology can be more readily resolved. It is also likely that we may abandon the use of overly general concepts such as alcoholism and drug addiction in favor of more refined and differential concepts. If in fact, as the Soviets contend, substance abuse can be strongly influenced or caused by such climatic conditions (e.g., cold temperature) or environmental factors (e.g., urban dislocation), and if differential treatments can be devised to appropriately deal with these external conditions, the addiction treatment field, both theoretically and clinically, will be vastly enhanced. Ultimately, both the Soviets and Americans seem to be moving in the same direction, namely that alcohol and drugs are not the cause of the problem, but rather a response to the problems confronted by the users.

Elsewhere I have remarked that "Addiction is a person problem, not a chemical problem. The ultimate resolutions will rest with demand reduction, not supply reduction. Abstinence without personal reorientation cannot be touted as a viable cure for addiction. The fact that some individuals (polydrug users) switch from one substance to another merely hallmarks that use is determined, in large measure, by the phenomenological experience that the drug creates for the user" (Lettieri, 1989).

It is encouraging to see the convergence in Soviet and American views of addiction. The papers in this volume highlight important theoretical developments in the thinking of Soviet addictionologists and presage new hope for effective treatments.

REFERENCE

Lettieri, D. J. (1989). *Substance abuse etiology. Treatments of psychiatric disorders. Vol. 2*. Washington, D.C.: American Psychiatric Association, pp. 1192-1202.

A REVIEW OF THE PROBLEM OF ALCOHOLISM IN SIBERIA. C. P. Korolenko and N. L. Botchkareva.

What is most impressive about this overview of alcohol problems in Siberia is its richness and complexity. In North America one is far more accustomed to encountering attempts to explain the emergence of such problems in relatively stark and simple terms (cf. Brower et al., 1989), with the current predilection being for biological and especially genetic (Petrakis, 1985) explanations. While such approaches have been appropriately criticized for their narrowness (Murray et al., 1983; Searles, 1988; Lester, 1988) they continue to emerge with monotonous regularity. Both direct personal contact and the occasional summary article in English (e.g., Anokhina, 1987) had led one to expect much the same from analogous Russian efforts, and indeed we have the confirmation from another paper in this series (Zavjalov) that there is a "most official" Soviet version of this monochromatic viewpoint.

Instead, what one finds in this paper is a vigorously flourishing eclecticism. In addition to psychological and biological factors it views such factors as climate, urbanization, industrialization, acculturation, population mobility, social relationships, economic and financial factors, recreational opportunities, and (by implication) many other elements as potentially critical in the development of alcohol problems. This refreshing and unexpected approach is strongly reminiscent of that taken by an experienced American epidemiologist:

> As an alternative to the common, static, unidimensional view of alcoholics as suffering a disease entity with a unitary cause, one can turn to a multifactored processes model. This way of thinking views every drinker as being at some stage of a dynamic, lifelong alcoholic process influenced by a multitude of weak, interacting social, psychological, and physical forces with no single factor, except alcohol, being necessary, and none at all being sufficient, to cause advancement in the process to the point of being labelled "alcoholic" or "problem drinker." From this viewpoint, the alcohologist's task of identifying the forces influencing the alcoholic process and untangling their complex interrelationships is much like that of the meteorologist's attempts to understand the processes called "the weather." (Mulford, 1982)

Those looking for a systematic and theoretical exposition of the viewpoint employed by the authors will not find it in this paper. However, another paper in this same series (Zavjalov) does provide such a perspective. Here, the framework evolved by this creative and industrious group of investigators is applied to understand the prevalence—said to be high—of alcohol problems in Siberia. Moreover, it is clear that the many factors these investigators see as relevant do not operate equally in every case or even upon every group. The implication of this heterogeneity for prevention and treatment efforts are thoroughgoing—no single approach will suffice. For example, the authors stress that treatment and prevention approaches must differ for immigrants to Siberia and for the native populations, since the factors impinging upon them are different.

Among the more fascinating of the possible variables considered is climate. That the unusual weather (and, to be sure, other) conditions occurring in an area like Siberia could produce unusual behavior was a theme often stressed by the poet laureate of the Yukon, Robert W. Service (1874-1958). For example:

> This is the Law of the Yukon, that only the strong shall thrive,
>   That surely the weak shall perish, and only the fit survive.
> Dissolute, damned, and despairful, crippled and palsied and slain,
> This is the Will of the Yukon — Lo, how she makes it plain!

Sam Magee, the protagonist of Service's best-known poem, welcomed his cremation as the first time he had been warm since leaving his native Tennessee.

As is usual, the more systematic exploration of variables known by perceptive artists like Service and others (Conrad, for example) to be important has lagged considerably. But is has been noticed. In one study, for example, a high positive correlation ($r = 0.79$) between average monthly temperature and the attrition rate from a drug-free therapeutic community over a two-year period was noted (Glaser, 1974). Although the possibility of a direct effect could not be dismissed entirely, it was felt the correlation was primarily due to the combination of increased activity in the illegal drug market and the decreased probability of apprehension by the authorities that occurred during the summer months.

Nevertheless, the examples are few and far between, and further exploration of climate as an influence on alcohol problems is certainly warranted. Given their acuity and vigor, our Siberian colleagues can perhaps lead the way. For example, by comparing alcohol problems in newly-arrived immigrants from less severe climates with such problems among those who relocate within similar climatologic areas in Siberia, they may be able to estimate the relative importance of mobility and climate as contributing factors.

One final comment: while the use of terms like "climate" and "acculturation" make it seem as if we are dealing with unitary phenomena when we speak of them, in fact each in its turn is composed of multiple variables. This, one supposes, is why Mulford (in the quotation above) speaks of the *processes* of the weather. If our factors themselves have factors, the ultimate phenomenon that we seek to explain — human behavior — must be very complex indeed.

Perhaps that is why it has taken us so long to understand it. Certainly that is why the present and future contributions of this able group of coworkers is so very welcome.

Frederick B. Glaser, MD, FRCP

REFERENCE

Anokhina, I. P., Ivanets, N. N., Burov, Yu. V. et al. (1987). Alcohol and alcohol problems research 13. U.S.S.R. *British Journal of Addiction, 82*, 23-30.

Brower, K. J., Blow, F. D., & Beresford, T. P. (1989). Treatment implications of chemical dependency models: An integrative approach. *Journal of Substance Abuse Treatment, 6*, 147-157.

Glaser, F. B. (1974). Splitting: Attrition from a drug-free therapeutic community. *American Journal of Drug and Alcohol Abuse, 1*, 329-348.

Lester, D. (1988). Genetic theory — an assessment of the heritability of alcoholism. In C. D. Chaudron & D. A. Wilkinson (Eds.), *Theories of alcoholism* (pp. 1-28). Toronto: Addiction Research Foundation.

Mulford, H. A. (1982). The epidemiology of alcoholism and its implications. In E. M. Pattison and E. Kaufman (Eds.) *Encyclopedic handbook of alcoholism*. NY: Gardner Press.

Murray, R. M., Clifford, C. A., & Gurling, H. M. D. (1983). Twin and adoption studies: How good is the evidence for a genetic role? In M. Galanter (Ed.), *Recent developments in alcoholism*. New York: Academic Press.

Petrakis, P. L. (1985). *Alcoholism: An inherited disease*. Washington, D.C.: U.S. Government Printing Office.

Searles, J. S. (1988). The role of genetics in the pathogenesis of alcoholism. *Journal of Abnormal Psychology, 97*, 153-67.

CLINICAL-PSYCHOLOGICAL APPROACHES TO ALCOHOL-ISM: MULTIPLE VERSIONS OF ALCOHOL DEPENDENCE. V. Yu. Zavjalov.

In Dr. Zavjalov's paper we are presented with terminology and approaches that are both familiar and unfamiliar. While the terminology used by Dr. Zavjalov differs from that in the Western literature, the search for new models that can help clinicians offer better and individualized treatment remains the same. Thus, the "clinical-psychiatric-oriented" (convergent) model appears to be a singularly-focused (unitary) model of alcoholism, comparable to our disease model. By contrast, the "clinical-psychological" (divergent) model appears to be a "multifocused" model that integrates not only "form" (psychological/sociocultural dimensions) and "stage" (classical psychiatry and neurology) — similar to our bio-psychosocial model — but also integrates the world views of the patient and therapist.

We have recently argued that all models have both advantages and disadvantages, but that one can maximize advantages while avoiding disadvantages through the integration of models (Brower, Blow, & Beresford, 1989). Dr. Zavjalov supports the need to be integrative. He writes: "An appropriate synchrony and harmony between . . . convergent and divergent manners of thinking . . . are the keystones of a new approach to alcoholism." Furthermore, the failure to integrate different models into clinical treatment is viewed as "dangerous: When a specialist has only one model of alcoholism . . . he/she appears to be in a very dangerous situation because they lose their flexibility and may thus encounter difficulty in relating to other human beings." Of course, the ultimate test of a model is its clinical utility: does it help us help our patients? As Dr. Zavjalov states, "Will the system work in psychotherapy, will it be useful for a specialist to help a patient change his or her behavior?" This question can only be answered by systematic research that assigns patients to different models of treatment and then assesses their outcome. In the meantime, therapists must be careful not to force all patients into one favorite model of treatment. Dr. Zavjalov eloquently argues for the need to consider the patient's point of view. In essence, one must determine which model the patient uses to understand his or her alcohol problem. Patients usually have their own ideas about why they drink and what will help them recover. As clinicians, we can either work with these ideas or clash with them, depending on how flexible our own models are. At the same time as we strive to understand our patients' motives for drinking, however, we must be careful not to collude with their rationalizations. If the patient believes their drinking is related to marital discord, for example, it does not follow that attention to marital issues will be sufficient treatment. Indeed, the marital problems may be caused by the drinking, rather than *vice versa*. Nevertheless, failure to pay attention to marital issues in such a patient — that is, failure to account for the patient's point of view — is an equal mistake. The marital issue, in this case, may provide the critical focal point for forming a therapeutic alliance with the patient for creating therapeutic leverage; whereas inflexibly insisting that the disease of alcoholism be the focal point may lead to a clash of "mismatch" between therapist and patient.

In conclusion, one must admire Dr. Zavjalov's attempt to break free of "the most official" model of alcoholism in the Soviet Union. At the same time, those of us in the United States must recognize the similar limitations of our own models of alcoholism, even if "freely" chosen.

J. Brower, MD
Department of Psychiatry
University of Michigan

REFERENCE

Browner K. J., Blow, F. C., & Beresford T. P. (1980). Treatment implications of chemical dependency models: An integrative approach. *Journal of Substance Abuse Treatment*; *6*, 147-157.

CLINICAL-PSYCHOLOGICAL APPROACHES TO ALCOHOL-ISM: MULTIPLE VERSIONS OF ALCOHOL DEPENDENCE. V. Yu. Zavjalov.

"What is the answer? [I was silent.] In that case, what is the question?" In her 1963 memoir *What is Remembered*, Gertrude Stein's devoted companion, Alice B. Toklas, recorded these as the last words of the expatriate American poetess. The exchange is worth pondering. Toklas knew that there was ultimately no reasonable answer to the question being posed by Stein, and Stein knew how to proceed in the absence of an answer.

Many of us feel what has been called "nostalgia for the absolute" (Steiner, 1974) so keenly we are unable to admit that answers to many important questions are not available. As a consequence we seize upon certain formulations, often simplistic or reductionistic ones, and cling to them desperately, going to the wall to defend them against any and all challenges. We insist that we know the truth, and cannot accept Sartre's definition of it as "that thing of indefinite approximation" (Sartre, 1956). Our position has been lampooned in a fantasy in which "the Ultimate Answer to Life, the Universe, and Everything" turns out to be 42 (Adams, 1983).

As Dr. Zavjalov points out, science is more than usually prone to this approach. Science is often construed by its practitioners as the search for the small number of universal truths that lie beneath the seeming diversity of existence. Some of the greatest triumphs of science have indeed been of this kind, such as the recognition of uniformities underlying the motions of the planets or the recognition that tabes dorsalis and general paresis were both, despite their very different clinical presentations, manifestations of syphilis. Science *is* this, then, but it is more than this. Science has to do with reality; and reality, while at times reducible to underlying principles, is at other times not so reducible. Reality is sometimes diverse:

> Natural historians insist that their work can only proceed beyond the anecdotal by continuous, repeated close observation—for there are no essences, there is no such thing as 'the chimpanzee.' You can't bring a few into a laboratory, make

some measurements, calculate an average, and find out, thereby, what chimpness is. There are not shortcuts. Individuality does more than matter; it is of the essence. You must learn to recognize individual chimps and follow them for years, recording their peculiarities, their differences, and their interactions. . . . I treasure this book [*The Chimpanzees of Gombe: Patterns of Behavior*, by Jane Goodall] for its quiet and unobtrusive proof, by iterated example rather than theoretical bombast, that close observation can be as powerful a method in science as the quantification of predictable behavior in a zillion identical atoms (we need both styles in their proper slots of our multifarious world). (Gould, 1987)

As does Stephen Jay Gould in the example above, Dr. Zavjalov also makes the point that these two views of reality are complementary, rather than antagonistic (cf. Blackburn, 1971). He indicates that persons manifesting problems that are associated with their consumption of alcohol are sufficiently alike that one can construct useful typologies (whether of alcohol problems per se or of aspects of such problems like motivation). But he also indicates that, at the same time, such persons are sufficiently different that therapy must be selected on a wholly individualistic basis. This approach is similar to that which Alvin Tarlov has seen as emerging in medicine generally:

Coming largely from behaviorists, a broadened paradigm of medicine has emerged out of the certain knowledge that one disease may be manifest among a group of patients in widely divergent ways and that illness as experienced by patients may be as highly individualized as fingerprints. The modern paradigm, not by any means intended by its protagonists to replace but rather to broaden prevailing thought, interacts disease with personal, social, and psychological factors to explain individual differences in illness. Despite face and experiential validity, the broadened paradigm has not achieved wide acceptance. (Tarlov, 1988)

That alcohol problems, although similar in some respects, are different in others, and that these differences are of great importance in matching individuals to treatment or treatments most likely to obtain a positive outcome, is the central point of Dr. Zavjalov's paper. It is also the central point of much current work on the treatment of alcohol problems in the United States, and particularly of a recent and comprehensive review of that treatment (Institute of Medicine, 1990). Yet despite this convergence, Dr. Zavjalov's paper came as something of a shock. Upon reflection, this reaction was not due so much to what was said as to who was saying it. That a Soviet psychiatrist working in Siberia should reach similar conclusions to those of an interdisciplinary committee drawn from all over the United States seems extraordinary. It is completely inconsistent with a view of Soviet psychiatry as the servant of its political masters and of Siberia as a punitive provincial backwater. Nor do the current and gratifying modifications in the structure and function of the Soviet state offer an understanding, since we are told that the present formulations are the most recent outgrowth of studies begun in the early 1970s.

Whatever the explanation, the convergence of viewpoints is exciting. We can only be grateful for the insights of our Soviet colleagues, and impatient to know more about their work. That they have learned from us is clear; one third of the references in this paper are to the American literature. Is there any paper in the alcohol field by an American author in which one third of the references are to the Russian literature? I do not think so. It is now time for us to learn from them. This issue of *Drugs and Society* is a signal step in that direction.

Frederick B. Glaser, MD, FRCP

REFERENCES

Adams, D. (1983). *The hitchhikers' trilogy*. New York: Harmony Books.
Blackburn, T. R. (1971). Sensuous-intellectual complementarity in science. *Science*, *172*, 1003-1007.
Gould, S. J. (1987). Animals and us. *New York Review of Books*, *34*(11), 23-24.
Institute of Medicine (1990). *Broadening the base of treatment for alcohol problems*. Washington, DC: National Academy Press.
Sartre, J. P. (1956). Portrait of the anti-semite. In W. Kaufmann (Ed.), *Existentialism from Dostoyevsky to Sartre*. NY: Median Books.

Steiner, G. (1974). *Nostalgia for the absolute*. Toronto: CBC Publications.
Tarlov, A. P. (1988). Introduction. in K.L. White, *The task of medicine: Dialogue at Wickenberg*. Menlo Park, CA: The Henry J. Kaiser Family Foundation.

CLINICAL-PSYCHOLOGICAL APPROACHES TO ALCOHOLISM: MULTIPLE VERSIONS OF ALCOHOL DEPENDENCE. V. Yu. Zavjalov.

Reviewing the work of a scholar whose cultural background is very different from one's own is a risky business at best. I take my cue from a colleague who recently visited the Soviet Union. He was surprised to find that psychiatrists in that culture are held in high esteem among medical practitioners while surgeons appear to inhabit the lower rungs of the medical hierarchy. A psychiatrist himself, he commented that the situation in America seems to be the exact reverse. These divergent social or cultural views of psychiatry bear on the present paper in that its Soviet author depicts a hierarchical vision of the problem of alcoholism in which the apogee is inhabited by psychiatry — more specifically psychiatric nosology — with a contribution of other disciplines resting in a "subordinated" role. These include the contributions of sociologists, psychologists, physiologists, and biologists. He then argues a case for a more egalitarian approach in which the disciplines of physiology, psychiatry, psychology and sociology all have contributions to make to the understanding of alcoholism that are ranked along side "common sense." In this view, he states a conclusion that is probably germane across all cultures: that each intellectual discipline has something to contribute to the understanding of the problem of alcoholism and, conversely, that no one discipline is likely to have all the answers. With consummate diplomacy, he then argues a case for using both the hierarchical and the egalitarian models of approaching alcoholism in a new synthesis that he titles the "clinical-psychological approach"; "clinical" and "psychological" here refer to the hierarchical and egalitarian modes respectively. In this sense, Dr. Zavjalov, writing from the Department of Psychiatry at the Novosibirsk Medical Institute, does an admirable job in arguing what I take to be an opening of the windows of Soviet psychiatry to let in the fresh breezes of new ideas and perspectives. In this effort, he serves the academic ideals common to all cultures and in the process evinces a richly humane approach to patient problems. When he discusses Bateson's view of the problems of intellectual rigor (in our culture symbolized by the nosological research of the last 20 years) as against the difficulties of "imaginative thinking" (roughly analogous to the emphasis on individual psychodynamics that psychoanalysis advocates in our culture), I found myself thinking that, despite all the difficulties of Stalinist and post-Stalinist Russia, Chekhov still lives.

Dr. Zavjalov argues for the importance both of intellectual "rigor" or the necessary effort of finding patterns and therefore prognosis in the problems of alcohol dependence, as well as for intellectual "imagination" or the necessity of understanding each patient's life as the primary avenue for assisting in healing and change. As the reader may surmise, many of the same struggles Dr. Zavjalov faces are to be found here in America, although with slightly different labels applied (Brower, Blow & Beresford, 1989). We have Dr. Zavjalov to thank for a clear view of the same struggle in his own country and culture, and for the understanding that humanity, perhaps irrespective of culture, faces the same challenge in understanding both the disease and the problems of alcohol dependence.

Thomas P. Bresford, MD
Department of Psychiatry
University of Michigan
and Scientific Director
University of Michigan Alcohol Research Center

REFERENCE

Brower, K. J., Blow, F. C., & Beresford, T. P. (1989). Treatment implication of chemical dependency models: An integrative approach. *Substance Abuse Treatment*, *6*, 147-157.

SOCIAL PSYCHOLOGICAL ASPECTS OF DRINKING BY YOUTH AND YOUNG ADULTS. A. S. Timofeeva and L. F. Perekrjostova.

This paper summarizes Timofeeva and Perekrjostova's views of "four developmental stages which are related to teenage alcoholism." Although the authors state that the identification of these stages resulted from their investigations, no details are given concerning the subjects employed or the procedures followed in those investigations. These views are useful, however, for comparison with current work on the stages of onset of alcohol and other drug abuse being conducted in the United States.

The first stage identified by the authors is "adaptation to alcohol," which begins with the first experience with alcohol, usually between the ages of 7 to 11 and usually in a family setting or with older schoolmates. According to the authors, the "appropriate education and pedagogical measures at this stage can stop youthful drinking." If these measures are not taken, the second stage begins about 2 to 3 months following initiation. The second stage is identified as "confirmation of stereotypes of alcohol behavior," during which time intoxication begins to be the goal and stronger ties are developed with drinking peers. Educational measures are still seen as adequate to stop the progression of alcoholism, but if appropriate measures are not taken in 2 to 12 months the third stage ensues. The third state is termed "psychological dependence on alcohol," during which time changes are experienced as a result of drinking (studying, family, hobbies, etc.). This stage is said to last for "several months to a year and a half." At this stage medical help is regarded as necessary in addition to educational measures. The final stage discussed by the authors is "physical dependence on alcohol" which includes loss of control, inability to abstain, and withdrawal symptoms. The appropriate intervention methods are not specified for this stage, but they are presumably similar to those for stage three.

The authors stress the need for early identification of and intervention with children at high risk for alcohol problems. A linkage between broad governmental social actions encouraging healthy lifestyles and the prevention of early alcoholism is regarded as necessary. Of tangential interest in the article is the mention of two epidemiologic studies conducted with Russian youth that suggest prevalences similar to those in the United States.

T. E. Dielman, PhD

ADDICTIVE BEHAVIOR IN WOMEN: A THEORETICAL PER-SPECTIVE. C. P. Korolenko and T. A. Donskih.

The paper presents information about 160 adolescent and adult women, from the ages of 15 to 60, drawing on detailed histories, descriptions of current behaviors, and some psychological testing. Although the authors don't describe how the sample was identified, it is likely that the data were collected from women seen for treatment or corrective intervention, since all of them appear to be experiencing problems with the use of alcohol or other drugs.

The authors begin by discussing some theoretical aspects of the concept of deviance, especially in the area of addictive behavior. They caution against viewing addiction too narrowly, and especially as primarily a form of "evil" behavior that represents moral failure; they assert that this "over-simplified" explanation of alcoholism results in narrowly focused, often highly emotional appeals to stop the deviant behavior and "prohibitionistic" social policies. Instead, the authors argue for a construction of addiction that has multiple forms and probably multiple causes. In this more complex formulation, prevention programs would require an understanding of the different forms of addictive behavior and the key elements in the backgrounds of persons who develop addictive behaviors.

Korolenko and Donskih note the difficulties that prohibitionistic approaches have had in other countries, and that variations in the outcomes of such policies in other countries were shaped by local social and cultural factors. The rest of the paper, however, does not explore the implications of the influence of culture for the Soviet Union or any of its regions. Instead, the authors' purpose appears to be to explicate a more complex understanding of "addictive disorders,'' suggesting an interaction between various factors. They note several types of initial motivation to change one's mental state, for instance, to relieve pain, to relax, to search for new and exciting sensations, to induce a dream-like state. They then describe briefly the development of psychological and physical dependence, and the complex of familial, psychological and social factors that can become involved in this process.

The authors initiate their discussion of women by describing the increase in the number of problem-drinking women in the USSR, from 5 to about 10%, but don't explore any reasons for this increase, except to note that misuse of alcohol has become a major problem within the USSR. They make no comparisons with comparable male data, or with information from women who are not experiencing problems with alcohol and other drugs. Instead, they focus on variations among women in their sample in order to explicate the complexity of the picture of addiction among women, and to begin to suggest some of the prevention and treatment strategies that may have relevance.

The purpose of this article thus appears to be less about explicating the circumstances of women in the USSR who experience problems with alcohol/other drugs, and more about using a sample of addicted persons who happen to be women. Although some aspects that are reported are key issues for women, or for a feminist analysis of women's status, the authors do not note or discuss these in that framework.

The data included appear to be predominantly self-reported family and personal histories, and, may be quite unreliable. Nonetheless, the profiles described are interesting and suggest different forms of, and routes to addictive problems. The profiles presented include 6 types based on family history, and two (apparently orthogonal) based on the relative importance of addictive or "anti-social" behaviors. The nature of the relationship between these two different typologies is not clear from the presentation.

What are not addressed in the paper are the factors that arise because those studied are women. All societies are gendered (shaped by gender-based assumptions and structures) in ways that have profound implications in any understanding of the circumstances of women, especially those labeled with some form of devi-

ant behavior. The authors don't raise these issues, nor do they com-
pare their data with what we know about women, alcohol and other
drugs in other countries. Questions that could be put to these data,
or that might help to guide future research on women and addiction
within the Soviet Union could include the following:

- In what ways is this particular society and community gendered? How do these processes influence how problems are
  defined similarly and differently for women than for men?
  How do they affect what is defined as deviant? How do they
  affect whether and how help is sought, and who is seen as
  useful helpers?
- What are the assumptions underlying treatment? In what ways
  are they affected by gender stereotypes? What are considered
  desirable outcomes for women, and how are these similar and
  different from those selected for men?
- Where and how are women experiencing problems with alcohol and other drugs identified? How do they find their way to
  treatment?
- What are the roles of family and peers in shaping later problems as well as adaptive coping? How are these similar and
  different for boys and girls?
- In what ways are women with problems with alcohol/other
  drugs perceived to be different from women not perceived to
  have those problems? What are the implications of these differences for prevention and case-finding?
- What are the implications of these (or other) subgroups among
  women for prevention and treatment? In what ways do cultural
  and class differences make a difference?
- Particular issues emerging as important for women in Western
  research suggest that the experience of sexual and family vio-
  lence may be particularly important in the etiology of problems with alcohol/other drugs. What is the relationship within
  the USSR of addictive problems with child sexual assault?
  Wife battering? Rape? The presence of these traumas suggests
  the need for different types of prevention and work on post-
  traumatic stress consequences.
- The data presented in this paper are very individually and psy-

chiatrically focused. The strengths and coping abilities of these women are not stressed. What social and societal factors have shaped their circumstances, and what survival mechanisms and skills are present?
—What other needs and problems do these women have that need attention (e.g., financial marginality, responsibilities for children, health concerns)?

Incorporating attention to these and other more gender-specific questions into future research should enable researchers, theorists, therapists, and policy makers to develop a better sense of the larger context of women experiencing problems with alcohol/other drugs within this culture. The current study begins to outline the complexity among women, and provides a substantial basis for the continuing study of a set of problems that include factors from the biological to the cultural-political. The authors are to be commended for this fine beginning.

Beth Glover Reed, PhD
University of Michigan
Social Work and Women's Studies

THE "RAPID COURSE OF DEVELOPMENT" OF EARLY ALCOHOLISM IN YOUNG PEOPLE. A. Dragun.

As the average age of those seeking treatment for alcoholism has dropped in recent decades, there has been increasing interest in the younger alcoholic/drug abuser. A review of the literature about the young male alcoholic (Gomberg, 1982) showed at least two authors who described, ". . . an acceleration of events," i.e., a telescoping of the developmental, phasic indicators of alcoholism (Hassall, 1968; Rosenberg, 1969). Obviously for the younger alcoholic, with fewer years to develop alcoholism there will be a telescoping of stages. Dragun's contribution is to analyze this telescoping and to point up differences *within* the younger age group. Starting with a group of 117 alcoholic males, aged 18 to 30, Dragun differentiates between those showing "a rapid course" – defined as manifestations of withdrawal within three years after onset – and those *not* showing such withdrawal. The two subgroups show some differences which may be of interest both to therapists and to preventers.

Young men who show "a rapid course" of the development of alcoholism report significantly more family history of alcoholism, paternal alcoholism, severe parental conflict, and significantly more "behavioral deviations" during their school years. Additionally, this group of young alcoholics remember their first intoxication experience better than do those not meeting the criterion for rapid course; 90% of the rapid-course group report "alcoholic euphoria" and positive memories of their first intoxication experience. This is interpreted by Dragun as a manifestation of, ". . . a rather high initial tolerance to alcohol."

The implications of several features of alcoholism among younger men for effective intervention have been discussed (Gomberg, 1986a), although these are drawn from a comparison of younger male alcoholics with an older group of male alcoholics. Dragun's findings suggest that it would be useful, working with young alcoholic men, to query about their first intoxication experience, the amount of alcohol consumed, and the use of "alcohol substitutes."

From a study of women alcoholics (Gomberg, 1986b), some related findings are of interest. Among the youngest woman alcoholics, aged 20 to 29, the time interval between first drink and first intoxication experience is significantly shorter than it is for the alcoholic women in their thirties and forties. The younger women alcoholics report blackout with the first intoxication experience significantly more often than do the other women, and when they are asked about feelings following first intoxication experience, the youngest women report significantly more often that they " . . . felt nothing," than do the older women. Perhaps these findings will inspire Dragun to include both men and women in future research on young alcoholics.

What impresses me, reading of young alcoholics in Novosibirsk, is the universality of acting-out behaviors with alcohol. There are reports from the United Kingdom, Canada, Hungary, Japan, South Africa and Australia about young alcohol-dependent persons, and these reports suggest that young people who turn to alcohol to solve their problems have much in common, regardless of where they are studied. I am also impressed by the good sense and truly multidisciplinary approach of this Novosibirsk investigator who seems to have no difficulty in presenting a point of view in which alcoholism involves, ". . . psychological and physical dependence," and no difficulty in seeing the influence of family history of alcoholism as including *both* genetic and psychosocial factors. Dragun's discussion, at the beginning of the paper, of the change from a community high consumption/few problems pattern to an increase in problem drinking related to migration, urbanization, and loss of traditional ceremonial drinking patterns, shows a breadth of understanding about alcohol problems which can include biology, personality and culture.

Edith S. Lisansky Gomberg, PhD

REFERENCES

Gomberg, E.S.L. (1982). The young male alcoholic. A pilot study. *Journal of Studies on Alcohol, 43,* 683-701.

Gomberg, E.S.L. (1986a) Some issues in the treatment of the young male alcoholic. *Alcoholism Treatment Quarterly, 3,* 109-118.

Gomberg, E.S.L. (1986b) Women and alcoholism: Psychosocial issues. National Institute on Alcohol Abuse and Alcoholism Research Monograph #16. *Women and alcohol: Health related issues.* (DHHS No. (ADM) 86-1139), 78-120.

Hassall, C. (1986) A controlled study of the characteristics of young male alcoholics. *British Journal of Addictions, 63,* 193-201.

Rosenberg, C.M. (1969) Young alcoholics. *British Journal of Psychiatry, 115,* 181-188.

THE "RAPID COURSE OF DEVELOPMENT" OF EARLY AL-
COHOLISM IN YOUNG PEOPLE. A. Dragun.

The purpose of the study reported in Dr. Dragun's paper was to
identify features differentiating alcoholic patients who exhibited a
more rapid onset of alcoholism from those who exhibited a more
"traditional" path to alcoholism. The study was carefully executed
and the results indicate useful directions for research predictors of
early onset of alcoholism. It also contains useful data for comparison with results in other countries.

The study began with 340 male industrial workers aged 18 to 30
years with a clinical diagnosis of alcoholism. Patients were excluded from the study if they were diagnosed as being only psychologically dependent (not physically dependent) on alcohol or if they
"showed signs of neuroses, psychopathic tendencies, serious physical or mental pathology, or brain damage." This screening process
resulted in a group of 117 patients who formed the basic study
group. These patients were divided into two groups, one (rapid onset group) which was composed of patients who evidenced alcohol
withdrawal symptoms within three years of the onset of regular
drinking ($N = 67$), and one (control group) which was composed of
patients who showed no withdrawal symptoms within three year of
the onset of regular drinking. The mean age of the patients in the
control group was slightly greater (23.7 years; range = 21-27) than
that of the rapid onset group (20.9 years; range = 19-26). The two
groups were similar with respect to age of onset of regular drinking,
educational level, and professional and marital status.

The two groups were compared with respect to a family history
of alcoholism or mental illness and other background factors, motives for drinking and drinking settings during their first contact
with alcohol, average length of time from the onset of regular drinking to the formation of symptoms of alcoholism, and personality
factor (as measured by the 16PF). The rapid onset group showed a
significantly greater prevalence of reports of a family history of
alcoholism, fathers' drinking, and intense parental conflict. A
greater percentage of the rapid onset group also reported mood alteration during their first contact with alcohol, retained reminiscences about their first contact with alcohol, an initial absence of

the vomiting reflex to overdoses of alcohol, and frequent conflict with parents and teachers while in school.

The analysis of differences in motives for drinking and the settings of the first contact with alcohol revealed basically the same patterns for both groups. The author states that the comparisons of the 16PF showed no overall profile difference between the two groups, but the mean scores of the rapid onset group were significantly lower on factors C and Q_3 and significantly higher on factors, L, O, and Q_4.

The comparisons on the mean length of time from the onset of regular drinking to the appearance of symptoms of alcoholism showed the rapid onset groups means to be shorter for all symptoms studied (loss of control, drinking bouts, alcohol amnesia, use of alcohol substitutes, and withdrawal syndrome). The means for the rapid onset group on these symptoms ranged from 1.4 to 3.5 years with standard deviations ranging from 0.1 to 0.3 years. The means for the control group ranged from 4.3 to 7.2 years with standard deviations ranging from 0.2 to 0.5 years. These findings should not come as a surprise in as much as withdrawal symptoms were used as the basis for forming the two groups, and withdrawal symptoms are correlated with the other symptom categories. Related to this, the author noted that the length of time to loss of control was significantly correlated with the length of time to the development of all of the symptoms of alcoholism, suggesting that early loss of control (1.5 to 2 years after the onset of regular drinking) may be a reliable criterion for the identification of drinkers at high risk of a rapid development of physical dependence on alcohol.

T. E. Dielman, PhD